tenminute
anti-ageing

ten minute
anti-ageing

ERICA BREALEY

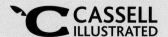
CASSELL
ILLUSTRATED

First published in the United Kingdom in 2003 by Cassell Illustrated
a division of Octopus Publishing Group Limited
2–4 Heron Quays, London E14 4JP

A CIP catalogue record for this book is available from the British Library

ISBN 1 84403 014 8

Editor: Victoria Alers-Hankey
Design by Austin Taylor
Jacket design by Jo Knowles
Photography by Paul Bricknell
Author photograph by Robin Farquhar-Thomson
Models for photography: Sandi Sharkey, Jo Robertson, Jan Mortimer, Erica Brealey.

Printed and bound in Italy

**If you are pregnant or if you have a medical condition
that could be adversely affected by exercise or have any
doubts about your health, consult a doctor before embarking on
any exercise programme.**

contents

introduction   6

1 understanding Ageing   8
why do we age?   10
what happens when we age?   10
preventable causes of ageing   12
what can we do to slow down
   the process?   13

2 the keys to staying young   14
reversing physical ageing   **16**
quit smoking   18
good sun sense   19
age-defying superfoods   20
anti-ageing supplements   22
staying in shape   26
keep active   29
menopause   32
hormonal help – HRT
   and the alternatives   34
beauty sleep   37
**reversing psychological
   ageing**   **38**
stretch your mind   40
a positive outlook   41
emotional health   42
spiritual fulfilment   43
meditation   44

3 ten minute anti-ageing strategies   46
face & hair   **48**
daily skin care   50
moisturizing facial massage   52
face masks   53
facial exercises   54
eyes   59
tooth care   61
hair and scalp   62
body   **64**
the body check   66
walking workouts   70
sun salutations   72
headstands and shoulderstands   74
gravity-defying exercises   82
hand care   108
feet   110
mind & spirit   **112**
mental exercise   114
deep relaxation   115
breath control   117
meditation techniques   121

golden rules   127

acknowledgements   128

introduction

*'Age, I do abhor thee;
Youth, I do adore thee'*
WILLIAM SHAKESPEARE

With a few choice words Shakespeare encapsulated an attitude to ageing that has changed little down the centuries. Far from revering the wisdom and maturity that come with age, we worship at the shrine of youth, our desire to look ever younger and more attractive, whatever the cost, generating a booming business for the purveyors of youth-enhancing, life-extending, beautifying elixirs.

The explosion of anti-ageing products promising to keep wrinkles at bay, firm saggy jowls, keep your mind sharp and your joints supple, has been accompanied by a dramatic rise in the number of people opting to have surgical and non-surgical cosmetic procedures. A new generation of techniques and treatments such as Botox and injectable fillers have opened up the market to people too squeamish to consider the scalpel, and the stigma attached to such procedures has all but disappeared. Millions routinely book a quarterly fix of injections to smooth furrowed brows and get rid of laughter lines, while women as young as their twenties throw Botox parties to ward off wrinkles before they even appear. From such beginnings it is but a short step to more invasive procedures.

It is easy to dismiss our obsession with youth and beauty as a symptom of social malaise; but the individual quest to prevent or reverse the signs of ageing is not just a question of vanity. In an ageist society looks really matter. Younger-looking, more attractive people earn more, make friends more easily and are treated with greater respect. No wonder so many of us, especially those in the public eye, feel under pressure to fix our appearance.

But do the cosmetics, cosmetic surgery and supplements industries really deliver on their promises of youth and beauty? Are expensive face creams, frozen Botoxed facial muscles, and pill-popping the answer to ageless ageing? And above all, are there any really effective alternatives?

The answer is an emphatic 'Yes'. Without resorting to cosmetic procedures, which carry the risk of side-effects, or going broke at your local cosmetics store, you can, with the help of tried-and-tested techniques and a little persistence, look not only healthy and attractive but much younger. Safe, natural alternatives such as facial exercises and massage may not produce instant results, but over the long term prove a highly effective way to firm and tone the facial muscles, taking years off your appearance. However, whether you opt for the high-tech approach or a natural one, or the best of both, there is much more to reversing the ageing process than acquiring a smooth, wrinkle-free face. With life expectancy rising sharply – over the last millennium the average lifespan in Britain has risen from 49 to 80 for women, and from 48 to 75 for men, and the lifespan of a typical woman in the US is estimated to be as high as 101 by 2070 – the emphasis is changing from how long you might live to the quality of life you might expect in your mature years.

Ten-Minute Anti-Ageing discusses the issues involved in the ageing process and the factors that contribute to it, and reveals the real secrets of enduring beauty and youthfulness. The ten-minute strategies offer quick – and sometimes instant – ways to make you look and feel younger and fitter, boost brain power and keep you young in spirit. The strategies also have a beneficial effect on health, preventing and reducing your risk of common conditions associated with ageing and increasing your chances of living to a ripe, productive and fulfilling old age.

It is never too late to take steps to avoid the preventable signs and symptoms of ageing, though the younger you start the better. There are no guarantees, but by devoting ten minutes a day – or even better two or three ten-minute blocks – to anti-ageing strategies you will be giving yourself the best possible chance of lasting good looks and of staying youthful in mind, body and spirit from maturity into old age.

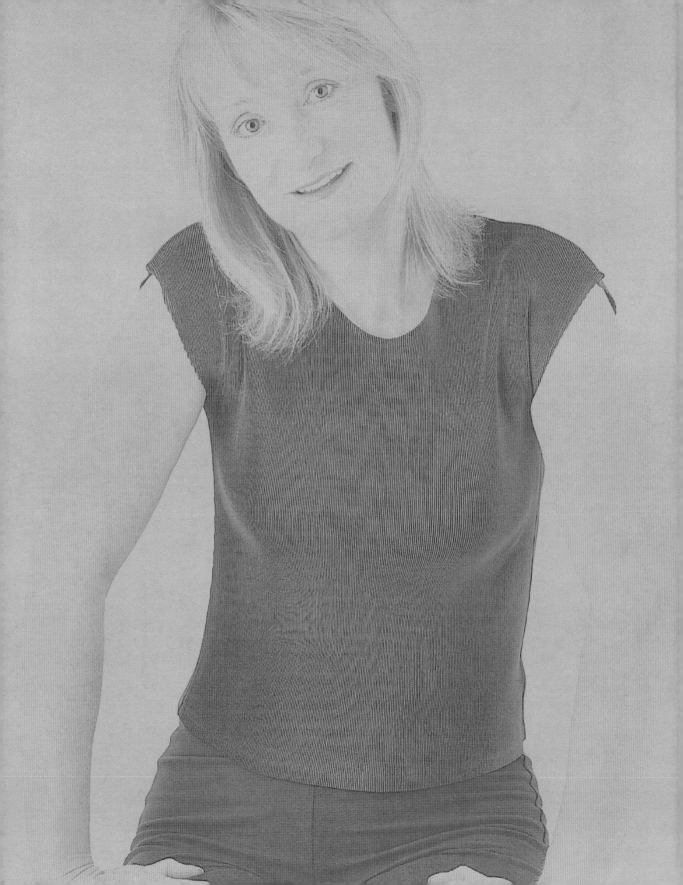

1

understanding
ageing

why do we age?

Even apart from the celebrity doyennes of the gossip pages whose looks invariably seem to defy their age, most of us can count among our family, friends and acquaintances the odd one or two whose looks and lifestyles totally belie their years, sometimes by decades. We watch with envy and amazement as they pass for students in their thirties, get taken for their kids' older brother or sister in their forties and fifties, build new lives and careers in their sixties or seventies, run marathons and travel the world in their eighties and nineties.

What is it about these people that keeps them looking young and vigorous, leading lives that defy all expectations, while the rest of us start counting grey hairs and wrinkles before we reach 40 and worry that we may be past our shelf-life once we hit it?

Looking and feeling younger than your years is partly down to luck, in the form of the genes your parents handed down to you. But though your genetic inheritance plays a part in determining your lifespan and how fast you age, their role in maintaining youthful good looks is a minor one – no more than a quarter of the total equation. It's the way you live your life that really makes the difference.

what happens when we age?

Inevitably physical changes, including changes in the skin, bones, joints, circulatory system, brain, nervous system and internal organs, occur with the passing of time, as the table on the opposite page illustrates. Mental faculties also decline with age.

Effects of ageing

BODY PART	HOW AGEING AFFECTS IT	FACTORS ACCELERATING AGEING
skin	Skin becomes drier, thinner and loses elasticity, causing it to slacken and wrinkles to form. Thread veins may become apparent. Skin bruises and tears more easily.	Smoking and exposure to cigarette smoke. Overexposure to strong sunlight. Excessive alcohol consumption. Pollution.
brain and nervous system	Memory is impaired and the ability to learn new skills weakens. Reaction times slow down.	Excessive consumption of alcohol and other recreational drugs. Activities and sports (such as boxing) that result in repeated blows to the head.
senses	All the senses tend to become less keen with age.	**Sight**: Prolonged use of VDUs without adequate breaks. **Hearing**: Overexposure to loud noise, such as very loud music or machinery. **Taste/smell**: Smoking
circulation	Harding of the arteries causes poor circulation and high blood pressure. This puts you at greater risk of heart disease and strokes.	Lack of exercise and obesity. Smoking and passive smoking. Poor diet, especially one high in fat. Excessive alcohol consumption.
muscles	Muscles shrink, often to be replaced by fat. Strength and flexiblity is lost.	Physical inactivity and lack of exercise. Starvation diets.
bones and joints	Bones become thinner and more brittle with age, a condition known as osteoporosis, leading to factures, reduced mobility, and loss of height. Post-menopausal women, and especially those who have gone through an early menopause, are particularly vulnerable.	Lack of weight-bearing exercise. Insufficient intake of calcium. Smoking. Heaving drinking. Obesity.

preventable
causes of ageing

As can be seen from the table on the previous page many of the causes of ageing are preventable, smoking leading the way as the single greatest preventable cause of premature ageing, ill-health and lost years of life.

The chart below shows the major preventable causes of physical ageing, ill-health and loss of life. It also illustrates the approximate extent to which each factor causes and accelerates ageing, both visible and internal.

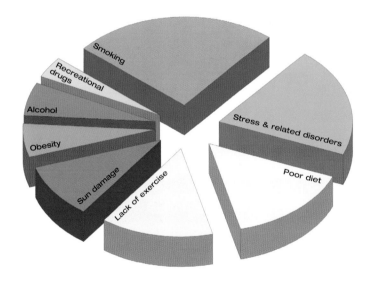

what can we do to slow down the process?

By avoiding smoking and over-exposure to the sun, minimizing stress and other factors that accelerate ageing, you can dramatically slow down the ageing process. However, research shows that looking after your mind is just as important as looking after your body when it comes to staying young and achieving a long life. By following the anti-ageing strategies described in this book, you can not only slow down but reverse many of the changes which come with the passage of time, and in doing so improve your overall health and your chances of a long life. A positive attitude pays huge dividends: optimists and people who engage in intellectual and creative activities aren't just younger in spirit. They live longer, happier lives.

Understanding what contributes to ageing and what you can do to counter it provides you with the tools you need to look great and feel in peak condition mentally and physically from your twenties to your sixties and beyond. When youthfulness is combined with the benefits that come with age – patience, wisdom, breadth of experience, and above all time – your mature years can be the happiest and most fulfilling of your life.

You don't have to give in to the negative aspects of age. Whatever your age, with a little effort and plenty of attitude, you can make it the prime of your life.

2
the keys to staying young

reversing
physical

As we have seen, people vary enormously in the rate at which they age, not just in terms of physical appearance and abilities, but in terms of the psyche too. For the sake of clarity and convenience this book treats the reversal of physical and psychological ageing separately, but the reality is that mind and body are two sides of the same coin, and anything you do to improve physical health is likely to have a positive impact mentally and emotionally. The connection between mind and body is never more apparent than when it comes to appearance. If you look good, you feel good. And how you treat your body is fundamental to maintaining young-looking skin and a good body.

Whether conscious or not, a healthy approach to life is one which people who look much younger than their actual age share. Very few of them smoke, and they tend to be physically active,

ageing

either because they take regular exercise or because their lifestyles involve a lot of physical activity. Their diet includes plenty of fresh fruit and vegetables and little convenience food, and a higher proportion are vegetarian than among the general population.

   If your lifestyle is not as healthy as it could be, take steps to improve it using the guidelines outlined over the next few pages. Begin by making simple adjustments to your diet and, if you are not in the habit of taking exercise, start now by walking whenever and wherever possible and incorporating one or more of the ten-minute exercise sequences into your daily routine. Be sure to get enough sleep too, and within weeks the years will begin to roll away from your face and body, and you will feel as well as look much younger.

quit smoking

If you are concerned about your appearance and you smoke, the best possible anti-ageing present you can give yourself is to stop. Apart from its harmful effects on your health and the role it plays in reducing life expectancy – knocking up to ten years off your life – smoking accelerates the rate at which skin ages, making smokers look older.

The reason for this is that smoking causes a reduction in collagen, the tissue that gives skin its elasticity, and weakens the skin's natural ability to renew itself. The result? Sagging and wrinkles. Research involving pairs of identical twins found that by middle age, a lifelong smoker's 'real' age was ten years older than their non-smoking twin's. Their skin was 40 per cent thinner, with more lines, more deeply etched.

the good news is that the benefits begin as soon as you kick the habit

The various health risks associated with smoking, such as lung cancer and heart disease, are well known. Smoking is even more dangerous for women than for men, increasing their risk of breast cancer, cervical cancer, early menopause and osteoporosis. The good news is that the benefits – and the list is endless – begin as soon as you kick the habit. You will look better, smell better, have more money in your pocket, and before long you will feel better and have more energy too. You will also live longer.

Stopping smoking is tough, and it can be scary. One of the main reasons why women in particular find it hard to give up is fear of weight gain. It is possible, though by no means certain, that you may temporarily put on a few pounds. But any weight gained should easily be lost unless you were below the correct weight for your body before quitting and used smoking to suppress your appetite. Other reasons – or excuses – include stress and anxiety. But the truth is that smoking cures nothing. It only creates problems. Your best defence against the deadly weed is resolve and will-power, but no one is saying it is going to be easy. If first attempts fail, try alternative remedies or seek professional help.

If you really can't quit, then be sure to offset (though don't kid yourself you can fully compensate for) the ill-effects of smoking with a diet high in antioxidants, found in brightly coloured fruit and vegetables, and vitamin C.

good sun sense

'Mad dogs and Englishmen go out in the midday sun'
NOEL COWARD

We all love to be in the sun – especially the English, who don't get nearly enough of it. It lifts our spirits and is beneficial to health. Vitamin D, which helps the body absorb calcium and is essential for the formation of strong bones and teeth, is produced in the body through the exposure of your skin to the sun's ultraviolet rays. As with most things, however, moderation is the key. Along with smoking, sun is the main cause of premature ageing of your skin.

How do you get the balance right? Although vitamin D is also found in foods such as oily fish, liver and egg yolks, exposure to sunlight is by far the most effective way to ensure the right levels of vitamin D in our bodies. Supplementation may sometimes be appropriate but excess can be toxic. Fortunately, the body's reserves of vitamin D can last for months, years even, and a little sun goes a long way. By exposing your hands and face to mid-morning sun for 15 or 20 minutes several times a week during the summer months, without applying sunscreen beforehand, your body should make enough vitamin D to last you throughout the year without damaging your skin. Alternatively protect your face and hands, and expose other parts of your body to the sun. The more skin you expose, the faster and the more vitamin D you will make.

To prevent premature ageing of your skin, invest in a good sunscreen with a sun protection factor (SPF) of at least 15 and apply it daily from March until November. Avoid or cover up in the midday sun. Damage done in your twenties will show up in your forties, but it is never too late to start protecting your skin.

Make a practice of wearing a hat and good quality sunglasses when out in strong sunlight. Wearing UV resistant sunglasses will protect your eyes from ultraviolet rays and prevent the formation of wrinkles around the eyes as a result of squinting into the sun.

> along with smoking, sun is the main cause of premature ageing for your skin

age-defying superfoods

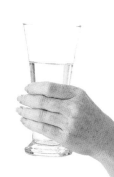

There is truth in the saying that we are what we eat. A glowing skin and good shape are the outward manifestation of inner health, which is dependent on how we nourish our bodies. A healthy, well-balanced diet is pivotal in holding back the ageing process and keeping wrinkles at bay.

To slow down ageing eat a balanced and varied diet, either as three square meals a day, or as several smaller meals spaced out across the day, and include on a daily basis:

- **plenty of fresh fruit or vegetables**, particularly brightly coloured ones rich in antioxidants (found in foods rich in vitamins A, C and E, such as tomatoes, peppers, carrots, broccoli, green leafy vegetables, watercress, apricots, oranges, papaya, berries). Antioxidants help prevent premature ageing of the skin by countering the production and effect of free radicals, the toxic by-products of the process by which the body converts oxygen into energy. Free radicals contribute to the visible signs of ageing – skin damage and wrinkles – and to the many other symptoms of age such as memory loss, heart and circulatory disorders, and some forms of cancer. Eat a minimum of five portions a day, raw or lightly cooked, choosing foods of different colours. Aim to build up to ten portions. Garlic and onions are also terrific anti-ageing foods which boost the immune system. If you find it difficult to digest so much fruit and veg in raw form, try juicing them or making soup.

- three or four helpings of **wholegrains** such as oats, brown rice, millet, rye, barley, which provide bulk and fibre, and are important sources of vitamin E, zinc and selenium (*see* page 21).

- one or two portions of **protein such as fish** (eat two or three portions of oily fish, such as salmon, tuna or sardines, a week as these are rich in fatty acids which keep your joints healthy and boost brain functioning), meat, cheese, eggs, non-genetically modified tofu or other soya products (particularly beneficial for women going through and post menopause) and beans.

- a handful of **mixed nuts and seeds**, good sources of vitamin E, zinc and selenium; linseed (flaxseed) is a particularly good source of essential fatty acids, also found in oily fish, while brazil nuts are an exceptionally good source of selenium.

- a **moderate amount of fat**, the best sources being vegetable oils such as olive oil, and fish oils (*see* above).

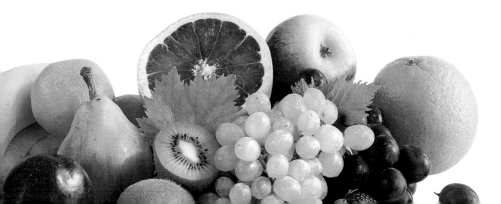

- the odd **glass of red wine**, which contains bioflavinoids, an antioxidant. A glass a day is anti-ageing and protects against heart disease; more than this accelerates the ageing process and leads to health problems such as liver and kidney disease.
- **tea**, especially green tea, is another good source of antioxidants, and protects against heart disease and some forms of cancer. But more than four or five cuppas a day, especially if drunk after mid-afternoon, keep you awake at night and raise stress levels.
- at least **two litres (eight glasses) of water**, and more if you live or work in a centrally heated or air-conditioned home or office. Drinking water regularly throughout the day keeps your skin healthy, hydrated and glowing by flushing out impurities and waste products from the system.

In addition to vitamins A, C and E, essential nutrients in an anti-ageing diet are:

- **zinc**, which boosts the immune system and works together with vitamins A, C and E and the minerals selenium and copper to slow down ageing. Good sources include wheatgerm, wholegrains, beans, fish and shellfish, sunflower seeds and brazil nuts.
- **selenium**, which like zinc plays an important role in slowing down and preventing the destruction of collagen and consequent formation of wrinkles, and other harmful effects of ageing. Brazil nuts are a very good source, along with garlic, onions, broccoli, wholegrains, fish and shellfish.
- **copper**, another important mineral for skin, protecting it from sun damage and helping it retain its elasticity. Good sources include prawns and other shellfish, nuts and beans.

Foods which accelerate the ageing process and should be cut out or cut down include:

- **refined sugar**, sugary foods and snacks, which weaken the skin's collagen causing it to lose elasticity and sag. Go for crunchy apples and raw vegetables such as celery and carrot sticks when you fancy a snack.
- **saturated fats** (animal fats and some vegetable fats, for example coconut oil) and hydrogenated trans fats found in biscuits, chips, and so on; fried foods.
- **fast foods**, convenience foods and other junk food. Fine once in a while, but these foods provide minimum nutrition and maximum calories.
- **excess alcohol** (*see* above).

anti-ageing
supplements

There is little doubt that the best way to get the vitamins and minerals your body needs is through a healthy diet rich in fruit and vegetables, the beneficial effects of which cannot be replicated in the form of pills. However, opinion is divided as to whether or not all our nutritional requirements can be met through diet alone. In an ideal world they should be, assuming you eat a balanced diet, and certainly supplements are no substitute for a high-quality, nutritious diet. On the contrary they are far more effective when taken in conjunction with a balanced diet. But while commercial considerations may lie behind some recommendations to supplement diet with vitamins, minerals, essential fatty acids and so on, many people benefit from appropriate supplementation, and supplements such as antioxidant vitamins can do you no harm.

The perplexing question is, what do you need and where do you begin? A bewildering array of herbal, vitamin and mineral, antioxidant and other supplements are available in the form of pills, powders, capsules and tinctures. Ideally you should consult a nutritional advisor before beginning a supplementation programme, but you are unlikely to experience any adverse reactions from self-supplementation if you stick to the recommended dosage of any particular supplement, and so long as you are careful to check the combined amount of vitamins A and D in any supplements you may take, as an excess of these vitamins can be toxic.

If your diet is not all it could be, or you feel under par, take a broad-spectrum vitamin and mineral supplement which will provide you with the recommended daily amount (RDA) of essential vitamins and minerals. Alternatively pick and mix as appropriate among the following anti-ageing supplements, but always consult your doctor first if you are pregnant, on prescription medication, or if you suffer from depression or epilepsy.

Antioxidants

Antioxidants are being hailed as the ultimate elixirs of youth, potent remedies against the ageing process in all its many forms, due to their role in destroying free radicals (see page 20). The following are some of the most effective:

• **antioxidant vitamins** including **vitamin A**, best taken as beta carotene, which boosts the immune system, keeps eyes moist and skin supple, dosage 15 mg daily; **vitamin C** which helps fight infections and boosts the production of collagen, dosage from 1000 mg in your twenties increasing by 500-mg increments to 3000 mg in your fifties; **vitamin E** which protects against premature ageing of the skin, disorders of the nervous system, memory loss, heart and circulatory system, and some forms of cancer, dosage from 200 IU in your thirties increasing by 100-IU increments to 400 IU in your fifties and beyond;

- **Pycnogenol** is a potent antioxidant which helps reverse and protect against ageing of the skin, helping the body to maintain and build collagen and elastin, which restores the skin's plumpness and elasticity, and also protecting against the formation of thread and varicose veins. Supplementation recommended for those over 30–35. Dosage from 30–100 mg a day.

- **alpha lipoic acid** is an antioxidant found naturally within the body which has been found to protect against diabetes and heart disease, and is thought to be particularly effective in reversing ageing when taken in combination with acetyl-L-carnitine (*see* below). Supplementation recommended for those over 45. Dosage from 100–200 mg a day.

the best way to get the vitamins and minerals your body needs is through a healthy diet

- **acetyl-L-carnitine** is another powerful antioxidant found naturally in the body. It improves brain function and memory, boosts energy levels and helps skin repair. Supplementation is recommended if you are over 45–50, and is said to be especially effective in combination with alpha lipoic acid (*see* above). Dosage 100–300 mg daily.

- **coenzyme Q10** is found naturally in the body and is essential for healthy skin. It also protects against heart disease and boosts brain function. Supplementation recommended from 30 onwards. Dosage 30–100 mg a day.

- **omega-6** and **omega-3 essential fatty acids (EFAs)** improve skin, boost brain power and energy levels, and generally fight the infections that generate free-radical activity and premature ageing. Although most people's diets are fairly rich in omega-6 EFAs, unless you eat oily fish or a handful of nuts and seeds on daily basis you are likely to be deficient in omega-3. Good sources of omega-3 are cod liver oil and docosahexaenoic acid (DHA). Dosage 100–400 mg a day.

B-complex vitamins

All the B vitamins are essential, protecting against heart disease, keeping the nervous system in good condition and allowing the release of energy into the body. **Folic acid**, part of the B complex, is especially important for women in their childbearing years as it reduces the risk of their unborn babies developing spina bifida. Vegans should consider supplementing with **B12**, as their diets tend to be low in it, causing depleted energy levels and fatigue. Low levels of **B6** can also be a cause of tiredness, as well as mood swings and depression. Dosage 200–400 mcg a day of folic acid, 20–400 mcg a day of B12, 10–100 mg of B6. Alternatively take a B-complex supplement as this will be correctly balanced in terms of the various B-complex vitamins.

Minerals

- **selenium** (*see* page 21), dosage 50–200 mcg a day.
- **zinc** (*see* page 21), dosage 10–50 mg a day.
- **calcium** is essential for building healthy bones and reducing the risk of developing osteoporosis; however, an excess can result in calcium deposits building up in the walls of the arteries. Supplementation recommended from mid-thirties. Dosage 500–800 mg a day depending on dietary intake.

Herbal help

Several herbs, including some used in everyday cooking – oregano, sage, rosemary and thyme – are known to have anti-ageing properties. Fresh and dried herbs for culinary use are less potent than herbs prepared for medicinal purposes and can be used freely in food preparation. Other helpful herbs include those listed on the opposite page, which may be taken in capsule, tablet or tincture form, dosage as recommended by the manufacturers or your nutritional therapist or herbalist. Always consult a medical practitioner if you have any chronic or serious health problems, if you are pregnant or breastfeeding, or are taking any prescription medicines as some herbs can interfere with the action of certain drugs. If self-medicating it is best to introduce one herb at a time and monitor your response to it, bearing in mind that it can take three or four weeks for effects to be felt. If you notice no improvement after two months, then the herb is not helping and there is no point in carrying on with it. Most herbs can be taken indefinitely without any adverse effects, but unless instructed differently by your therapist, you are advised to take a break for at least a month every three to six months.

- **black cohosh** has an oestrogenic effect and is often used as an alternative to hormone replacement therapy (HRT). It relieves menopausal symptoms such as hot flushes, night sweats and vaginal dryness. Combining black cohosh with St John's wort (see below) has been found as effective as HRT in countering unwelcome symptoms for many women.
- **dong quai** is often referred to as the female ginseng owing to its energy-boosting effects. Its benefits include relief from menopausal symptoms such as hot flushes, alleviation of joint pain and protection against osteoporosis. Avoid during pregnancy.
- **ginkgo biloba** is well known for improving memory, but also brings numerous other health benefits. It increases blood flow to the extremities – brain, hands and feet – boosting brain function and helping to prevent cold hands and feet.
- **ginseng** helps counter stress and boosts immunity and energy levels.
- **red clover** mimics the effects of oestrogen and is another herb used as an alternative to HRT to relieve the symptoms of menopause such as hot flushes and mood swings.
- **sage** is an oestrogenic and helps alleviate menopausal symptoms, especially hot flushes. It is also rich in antioxidants and so protects against premature ageing. Avoid during pregnancy.
- **St John's wort (hypericum)** has been shown to be as effective as Prozac in treating mild to moderate depression. It can also help with irritability, hot flushes, disturbed sleep and low sex drive. Consult your doctor before taking this herb if you are taking anticoagulant drugs such as warfarin, prescription antidepressants or if you are on the pill.

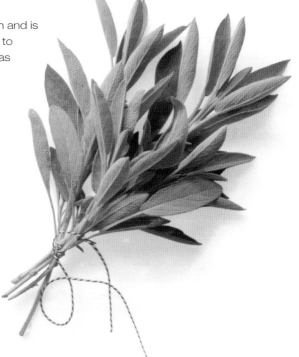

staying in shape

Although a few extra pounds can make women look younger, resulting in attractive curves, plumping out the skin and stopping it from sagging, with age excess weight can have the reverse effect. Once you hit your middle years, and especially after the menopause, fat tends to settle in the wrong places. This makes you look more shapeless than curvy, with the added disadvantages that weight gets more difficult (but not impossible!) to lose as your metabolism slows down, and you tend to lose it from the wrong places, so everything drops.

Slim people not only look younger – we associate youth with slender, shapely bodies – they are healthier and live longer too. Excess weight increases your risk of suffering from potentially fatal illnesses including heart attacks, high blood pressure and diabetes. Whatever your age, if you are overweight, take steps to get into shape now.

The body mass index (BMI) is the most commonly used guide to acceptable weight ranges for any given height, and is widely used for assessing levels of overweight and obesity, underweight and emaciation.

Calculating your BMI:

$$BMI = \frac{\text{weight in kilograms}}{(\text{height in metres x height in metres})}$$

Example:

Weight =	9 stone 3 pounds	= 58.5 kilograms
Height =	5 feet 5 inches	= 1.65 metres
BMI =	$\frac{58.5}{(1.65 \times 1.65)}$	= 21.5

You do not, however, need any mathematical skills to work out your BMI. The table will do this for you.

BMI ranges:

below 15: *emaciated*
16 – 19: *underweight*
20 – 25: *healthy*
26 – 30: *overweight*
above 30: *obese*

The Body Mass Index (BMI) Table

HEIGHT (Feet and Inches)

WEIGHT (Kilograms)

kg	4'6"	7"	8"	9"	10"	11"	5'0"	1"	2"	3"	4"	5"	6"	7"	8"	9"	10"	11"	6'0"	1"	2"	3"	4"	5"	6"	7"
110	59	57	55	53	51	50	48	46	45	43	42	41	40	38	37	36	35	34	33	32	31	31	30	29	28	28
109	59	57	55	53	51	49	48	46	45	43	42	40	39	38	37	36	35	34	33	32	31	30	29	29	28	27
108	58	56	54	52	51	49	47	46	44	43	41	40	39	38	37	36	34	34	33	32	31	30	29	28	28	27
107	58	56	54	52	50	48	47	45	44	42	41	40	38	37	36	35	34	33	32	31	31	30	29	28	27	27
106	57	55	53	51	50	48	46	45	43	42	41	39	38	37	36	35	34	33	32	31	30	29	29	28	27	27
105	57	55	53	51	49	47	46	44	43	42	40	39	38	37	36	35	34	33	32	31	30	29	28	28	27	26
104	56	54	52	50	49	47	45	44	42	41	40	39	37	36	35	34	33	32	31	31	30	29	28	27	27	26
103	56	54	52	50	48	47	45	43	42	41	39	38	37	36	35	34	33	32	31	30	29	29	28	27	26	26
102	55	53	51	49	48	46	45	43	42	40	39	38	37	36	35	34	33	32	31	30	29	28	28	27	26	26
101	55	53	51	49	47	46	44	43	41	40	39	37	36	35	34	33	32	31	30	30	29	28	27	27	26	25
100	54	52	50	48	47	45	44	42	41	40	38	37	36	35	34	33	32	31	30	29	29	28	27	26	26	25
99	54	52	50	48	46	45	43	42	40	39	38	37	36	35	34	33	32	31	30	29	28	27	27	26	25	25
98	53	51	49	47	46	44	43	41	40	39	38	36	35	34	33	32	31	30	30	29	28	27	27	26	25	24
97	52	51	49	47	45	44	42	41	40	38	37	36	35	34	33	32	31	30	29	28	28	27	26	26	25	24
96	52	50	48	47	45	43	42	41	39	38	37	36	35	34	33	32	31	30	29	28	27	27	26	25	25	24
95	51	49	48	46	44	43	41	40	39	38	36	35	34	33	32	31	30	29	29	28	27	26	26	25	24	24
94	51	49	47	46	44	42	41	40	38	37	36	35	34	33	32	31	30	29	28	28	27	26	25	25	24	24
93	50	48	47	45	43	42	41	39	38	37	36	35	33	32	32	31	30	29	28	27	27	26	25	24	24	23
92	50	48	46	45	43	42	40	39	38	36	35	34	33	32	31	30	29	29	28	27	26	26	25	24	24	23
91	49	47	46	44	43	41	40	38	37	36	35	34	33	32	31	30	29	28	27	27	26	25	25	24	23	23
90	49	47	45	44	42	41	39	38	37	36	34	33	32	31	30	30	29	28	27	26	26	25	24	24	23	23
89	48	46	45	43	42	40	39	38	36	35	34	33	32	31	30	29	28	28	27	26	25	25	24	23	23	22
88	48	46	44	43	41	40	38	37	36	35	34	33	32	31	30	29	28	27	27	26	25	24	24	23	23	22
87	47	45	44	42	41	39	38	37	36	34	33	32	31	30	29	29	28	27	26	26	25	24	24	23	22	22
86	47	45	43	42	40	39	38	36	35	34	33	32	31	30	29	28	27	27	26	25	25	24	23	23	22	22
85	46	44	43	41	40	38	37	36	35	34	33	32	31	30	29	28	27	26	26	25	24	24	23	22	22	21
84	45	44	42	41	39	38	37	35	34	33	32	31	30	29	28	28	27	26	25	25	24	23	23	22	22	21
83	45	43	42	40	39	37	36	35	34	33	32	31	30	29	28	27	27	26	25	24	24	23	22	22	21	21
82	44	43	41	40	38	37	36	35	33	32	31	30	30	29	28	27	26	25	25	24	23	23	22	22	21	21
81	44	42	41	39	38	37	35	34	33	32	31	30	29	28	27	27	26	25	24	24	23	22	22	21	21	20
80	43	42	40	39	37	36	35	34	33	32	31	30	29	28	27	26	26	25	24	23	23	22	22	21	21	20
79	43	41	40	38	37	36	34	33	32	31	30	29	28	28	27	26	25	25	24	23	23	22	21	21	20	20
78	42	41	39	38	36	35	34	33	32	31	30	29	28	27	26	26	25	24	24	23	22	22	21	21	20	20
77	42	40	39	37	36	35	34	33	31	30	29	29	28	27	26	25	25	24	23	23	22	21	21	20	20	19
76	41	40	38	37	36	34	33	32	31	30	29	28	27	27	26	25	24	24	23	22	22	21	21	20	20	19
75	41	39	38	36	35	34	33	32	31	30	29	28	27	26	25	25	24	23	23	22	21	21	20	20	19	19
74	40	39	37	36	35	33	32	31	30	29	28	27	27	26	25	24	24	23	22	22	21	21	20	19	19	19
73	39	38	37	35	34	33	32	31	30	29	28	27	26	25	25	24	23	23	22	21	21	20	20	19	19	18
72	39	38	36	35	34	33	31	30	29	28	28	27	26	25	24	24	23	22	22	21	21	20	19	19	18	18
71	38	37	36	34	33	32	31	30	29	28	27	26	26	25	24	23	23	22	21	21	20	20	19	19	18	18
70	38	36	35	34	33	32	31	30	29	28	27	26	25	24	24	23	22	22	21	21	20	19	19	18	18	18
69	37	36	35	33	32	31	30	29	28	27	26	26	25	24	23	23	22	21	21	20	20	19	19	18	18	17
68	37	35	34	33	32	31	30	29	28	27	26	25	24	24	23	22	22	21	21	20	19	19	18	18	17	17
67	36	35	34	32	31	30	29	28	27	26	26	25	24	23	23	22	21	21	20	20	19	19	18	18	17	17
66	36	34	33	32	31	30	29	28	27	26	25	24	24	23	22	22	21	20	20	19	19	18	18	17	17	16
65	35	34	33	31	30	29	28	27	27	26	25	24	23	23	22	21	21	20	20	19	19	18	18	17	17	16
64	35	33	32	31	30	29	28	27	26	25	25	24	23	22	22	21	20	20	19	19	18	18	17	17	16	16
63	34	33	32	31	29	28	28	27	26	25	24	23	23	22	21	21	20	20	19	18	18	18	17	17	16	16
62	34	32	31	30	29	28	27	26	25	25	24	23	22	22	21	20	20	19	19	18	18	17	17	16	16	15
61	33	32	31	30	29	28	27	26	25	24	23	23	22	21	21	20	19	19	18	18	17	17	16	16	16	15
60	32	31	30	29	28	27	26	25	25	24	23	22	22	21	20	20	19	19	18	18	17	17	16	16	15	15
59	32	31	30	29	28	27	26	25	24	23	23	22	21	21	20	19	19	18	18	17	17	16	16	16	15	15
58	31	30	29	28	27	26	25	24	24	23	22	22	21	20	20	19	19	18	17	17	17	16	16	15	15	14
57	31	30	29	28	27	26	25	24	23	23	22	21	21	20	19	19	18	18	17	17	16	16	15	15	15	14
56	30	29	28	27	26	25	24	24	23	22	21	21	20	20	19	18	18	17	17	16	16	16	15	15	14	14
55	30	29	28	27	26	25	24	23	22	22	21	20	20	19	19	18	18	17	17	16	16	15	15	14	14	14
54	29	28	27	26	25	24	24	23	22	21	21	20	19	19	18	18	17	17	16	16	15	15	15	14	14	13
53	29	28	27	26	25	24	23	22	22	21	20	20	19	18	18	17	17	16	16	16	15	15	14	14	14	13
52	28	27	26	25	24	23	23	22	21	21	20	19	19	18	18	17	17	16	16	15	15	14	14	14	13	13
51	28	27	26	25	24	23	22	22	21	20	20	19	18	18	17	17	16	16	15	15	15	14	14	13	13	13
50	27	26	25	24	23	23	22	21	20	20	19	19	18	17	17	16	16	16	15	15	14	14	14	13	13	12
49	26	26	25	24	23	22	21	21	20	19	19	18	18	17	17	16	16	15	15	14	14	14	13	13	13	12
48	26	25	24	23	22	22	21	20	20	19	18	18	17	17	16	16	15	15	14	14	14	13	13	13	12	12
47	25	24	24	23	22	21	21	20	19	19	18	17	17	16	16	15	15	15	14	14	13	13	13	12	12	12
46	25	24	23	22	22	21	20	19	19	18	18	17	17	16	16	15	15	14	14	13	13	13	12	12	12	11
45	24	23	23	22	21	20	20	19	18	18	17	17	16	16	15	15	14	14	14	13	13	13	12	12	12	11
44	24	23	22	21	21	20	19	19	18	17	17	16	16	15	15	14	14	14	13	13	13	12	12	12	11	11

HEIGHT (Metres): 1.36 · 1.40 · 1.44 · 1.48 · 1.52 · 1.56 · 1.60 · 1.64 · 1.68 · 1.72 · 1.76 · 1.80 · 1.84 · 1.88 · 1.92 · 1.96 · 2.00

WEIGHT (Stones and Pounds) — right-hand scale markers:

- 17st / 238lb
- 7lb
- 16st / 224lb
- 7lb
- 15st / 210lb
- 7lb
- 14st / 196lb
- 7lb
- 13st / 182lb
- 7lb
- 12st / 168lb
- 7lb
- 11st / 154lb
- 7lb
- 10st / 140lb
- 7lb
- 9st / 126lb
- 7lb
- 8st / 112lb
- 7lb
- 7st / 98lb

Although it is a useful guide, the body mass index does not tell us the whole story. It does not, for example, take into account body types, If you have a petite frame, you are likely to be overweight and out of shape at a BMI of 25, while at the other end of the scale some highly fit people – usually men – can fall into the obese category without being either overweight or obese. This is because muscle weighs more than fat, so those with well-developed muscles tend to score relatively highly on the scale.

How fat is distributed is equally important for your health and youthful looks as where you tip the scales. Too much around the middle (more than 80 cm/32 inches for women, 94 cm/37 inches for men) means you definitely need to take action.

Anti-ageing weight loss

If you want to lose weight and maintain your weight loss, you need to adopt a healthy and satisfying pattern of eating for the rest of your life. Avoid crash diets or faddy diets. They usually result in yo-yo weight – the fast route to ageing, saggy skin – and put you at a higher risk of developing osteoporosis. By following the eating plan on pages 20-21 and taking regular exercise (see pages 30–31) you will almost certainly lose weight if you have excess fat to lose.

Other tips for weight loss include:
• eating little and often – research shows that people who eat six smaller meals a day weigh less than those who eat the same number of calories in one or two sittings
• drinking a glass of water before beginning your meal and/or having soup or a salad as a starter. It will fill you up and mean you eat less of your main course
• eating more slowly. This allows time for the body to register and send out a signal when its hunger is satisfied – and gives you a chance to absorb the message
• binning the kids' leftovers before you're tempted

keep active

Keeping active is not only the most significant factor in promoting all-round physical and mental health, it really can turn back the clock and reverse the ageing process. There has been a shift away from the traditional recommendation of 30 minutes of vigorous exercise at least three times a week, to taking more moderate exercise, more frequently. Ideally we should all accumulate 20 or 30 minutes of moderate physical activity most days, but this can be split up into ten-minute sessions. Ten minutes' aerobic exercise, vigorous enough to make you slightly out of breath, will not only tone your muscles, it will make your skin glow and make you look younger.

Where your muscles are concerned that old cliché, use it or lose it, really does apply. After your mid-to late twenties, when muscle mass and bone density reach their peak, you will lose muscle at a rate of more than half a pound a year, and by as much five or six pounds a year with advancing age, without exercise. This impacts on your bones and leads to loss of strength and endurance, low energy levels and, on the looks front, makes you flabby and untoned. You are likely to gain weight too because muscle wastage lowers your metabolic rate, so you will need to eat less to stay the same weight. Physical inactivity accelerates the ageing process and puts you at a much higher risk of suffering a heart attack, circulatory problems, disability and osteoporosis. A sedentary, inactive lifestyle can double a woman's risk of hip fracture and increases the likelihood of an early old age spent hunched up and bent double. So ditch the car and get moving.

The younger you begin to take regular exercise – accumulating at least an hour and a half of exercise a week, preferably more – the better. But the good news is that it is never too late to start, or to enjoy the benefits of an exercise regime and reverse the signs and symptoms of physical ageing. In fact, the older you are, the more likely you are to notice the improvements. One study on people in their seventies showed a walking programme to reverse 22 years of declining lung capacity in 22 weeks, while people in their fifties and even sixties can regain the fitness and tone of a 20-year-old. Strength can be improved even in extreme old age, and the benefits will not be confined to your body.

If the thought of exercise fills you with dread, find alternative ways to keep active doing something you enjoy. Try putting on some disco music and dance to it for ten minutes. Take a brisk ten-minute walk around your local park. Or break yourself in gently by wandering around an art gallery or museum. Once your body gets into the habit of moving you will look and feel so much better you won't want to stop.

Exercise and the mind

Just as it tones and strengthens your muscles, moderate exercise appears to have a similar effect on your mind, probably due to the increased flow of blood to the brain. Moderate exercise has also been found to boost memory and brain power, improving for example the ability to plan and organize, and to reverse symptoms of mental decline associated with ageing, perhaps even delaying the onset of Alzheimer's. Exercise also raises energy levels, lowers stress levels, lifts depression, builds self-confidence and self-esteem, helps you sleep and, due to the endorphins released, makes you feel happier and more positive.

Exercise and your age

Age is no barrier to exercise, and certainly no excuse to avoid it, though needs and focus may vary with age.

• **Twenties** Exercise is often low on the list of priorities in your twenties, but by developing good habits now you can lay down the foundations of a long and youthful life. Ideally every exercise programme should include: *aerobic activity* such as running, cycling, ashtanga yoga and swimming for cardiovascular and respiratory health, and to strengthen muscles. *weight-bearing exercise* – exercise that involves impact between your feet and the floor – such as brisk walking, running or skipping, to build strength and increase bone density. *stretching exercise* such as dancing, gymnastics or any form of yoga to increase suppleness and flexibility.

• **Thirties** This is likely to be one of the most challenging stages of your life, juggling a career in full swing with the demands of a young family. Regular exercise as in your twenties will keep you fit and toned, keep stress at bay and increase your energy levels. If time is of the essence, the key is little and often. Walk or cycle whenever you can rather than taking the car or public transport, and practise at least one ten-minute exercise sequence, such as the sun salutations (*see* pages 72–73) every day. Women, especially during pregnancy and following childbirth, should do pelvic floor exercises daily.

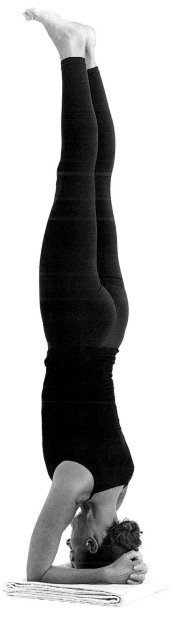

• **Forties** In the absence of appropriate weight-bearing exercise, bone density starts to decrease in earnest, particularly in women in the run-up to the menopause. Continue or begin a combination of aerobic, weight-bearing and stretching exercise as before. Weight resistance training increases muscle strength, which supports and protects your bones, and also prevents undue loss of bone. Aerobic activity ensures that oxygen-rich blood circulates to your skin, increasing radiance and making you look younger.

• **Fifties and beyond** Loss of bone density accelerates in women after the menopause, and by 60 most women only have two-thirds the muscle they had at 20. The more exercise you do before you hit 60, the younger and healthier you will look and feel in your sixties. If you are not already in the habit of regular exercise, begin with ten minutes' walking every day, building up to twice a day, and ten minutes of gentle stretching exercise such as yoga or Pilates at least three times a week to keep you supple. If you stick with it you will build up strength and flexibility, but avoid overdoing it, especially if you are overweight or have high blood pressure.

Yoga

Hatha yoga – the branch of yoga devoted to physical postures and breathing exercises – deserves special mention in any anti-ageing book as one of the best overall anti-ageing therapies on the planet. There is a wide range of styles, from gentle and meditative to the physically demanding ashtanga, and many of the exercises in Part 3 are based on classic yoga postures. Regular practice brings immense benefits both mentally and physically, developing strength, stamina and flexibility, boosting the immune system, increasing energy levels, calming the mind and increasing concentration and of course relieving stress. There is no age limit: you can begin yoga at 15, 50 or at 80. Yoga works on the whole system, internal and external, restoring and maintaining the elasticity of the spine, and breathing flexibility and life into neglected parts of the body which have lost their youthful suppleness.

menopause

Menopause, strictly speaking, is the point in time when a woman has her final menstrual period, normally between the ages of 45 and 55. The reality, however, is that the menopause is experienced as a period of transition, physically and psychologically, which can last several years. It is a time of shifting hormone levels triggered by the decrease in the production of eggs by the ovaries as a woman's childbearing years draw to a close and she enters a new phase of her life.

Since it marks the end of a woman's reproductive life, the menopause is an undeniable reminder of the passage of time and the fact of physical ageing. In the long term the major concerns for post-menopausal women are their increased risk of coronary heart disease and strokes, which now becomes comparable to the risk factor for a man, and of osteoporosis (loss of bone density and increasing brittleness of the bones). In the meantime, as a woman approaches menopause she may temporarily experience irregular or very heavy periods, increased premenstrual tension and migraines as progesterone levels decrease. Classic but passing symptoms due to declining oestrogen levels as a woman goes through the menopause include hot flushes (by far the most common symptom, experienced to some degree by most women in the West) and night sweats, vaginal dryness and loss of libido, headaches and migraines, fuzzy thinking and memory loss, and mood swings. Other symptoms reported are irritability, tearfulness and depression, though these may have as much to do with lifestyle and general ageing as they do with fluctuating hormones.

Just as women react differently to changing hormone levels during adolescence and pregnancy, so each woman's experience of menopause is unique. Women who go through an early menopause, or who are very stressed, are likely to get more severe symptoms, as are women who are plunged into an abrupt menopause induced by surgery or medical treatment for illnesses such as cancer. More fortunate women have few if any unwelcome symptoms, and certainly nothing that warrants a trip to the doctor or alternative-health practitioner. Following the advice in this section – regular exercise, a healthy diet and appropriate nutritional supplements, not smoking and a moderate alcohol intake, taking time to relax and a positive outlook – will maximize your chances of an easy transition, but it is a complex process, and there are no guarantees. If your symptoms are causing you distress or discomfort, explore herbal remedies, diet and nutritional supplements that will help support the change or consider HRT – see overleaf. If you have decided against taking hormones, it can help to remember that unwanted symptoms will pass, and once you emerge from the transition you are likely to discover renewed energy and zest for life.

For all women, however they experience it, the menopause marks a change of life. Whether it unfolds as a passage towards greater wisdom, fulfilment and inner strength, or whether it marks the beginning of a gradual decline, is strongly influenced by your expectations of and approach to menopause. A good diet and regular, appropriate exercise – aerobic for your heart and weight-bearing to protect your bones – will reduce your risk of heart attacks and osteoporosis; exercising your mind – keeping intellectually active and pursuing your interests – nurtures your brain and helps preserve memory; and an optimistic attitude gives you the impetus to make positive changes in your life. Rather than seeing the menopause simply as a loss of youth, sexuality and fertility, look for the opportunities it offers, such as the chance to express creativity in other ways than giving birth and rearing children. For many women the post-menopausal years are the happiest and most fulfilling of their lives. To some the change of life comes as a call to re-examine their lives and take it in new directions. To others it is about getting in touch with the spirit, discovering the inner realms and contemplating the eternal.

hormonal help – HRT and the alternatives

An individually tailored programme which may or may not include hormone replacement therapy can go a long way towards easing both the physical and psychological symptoms of the menopause.

Hormone Replacement Therapy (HRT)

HRT was long regarded by the medical establishment as something of a panacea – the best 'cure' for the troublesome symptoms of menopause such as hot flushes and night sweats, and its favourite preventative medicine for the diseases – in particular heart disease, osteoporosis and Alzheimer's – that can follow in its wake. Women are attracted to HRT not just to deal with the symptoms of menopause and to counter the long-term effects of hormonal changes, however. The HRT marketing machine has touted the drug as a veritable elixir of youth and convinced women it will keep them looking and feeling young and sexy, with glowing skin, lustrous hair and an inexhaustible supply of energy.

HRT comes in a variety of forms and formulas, most often as a combination of oestrogen and progesterone, though progesterone may be omitted in women who have had a hysterectomy, and can be taken by means of pills, implants, patches, vaginal creams, coils, gels or pessaries. At the time of writing between a third and a fifth of all women over 50 in the UK take some form of HRT and many women seem to do well and feel good on it. But HRT has been controversial since it was introduced and claims once made for the drug are now in question. HRT can have unwelcome side-effects and, as with all drugs, there are risks attached to taking it.

That HRT protects against osteoporosis is fairly uncontroversial, and for women who are at risk of the disease – because, for example, they have gone through an early menopause, suffered from anorexia, have a family history of the disease – it has traditionally been the first choice of treatment. However, the drug protects against loss of bone density only so long as you take it, with bone thinning in women who stop taking HRT catching up within a few years to what it would have been had they never taken the drug. Since half of all women prescribed HRT stop taking it within a year because of its unpleasant side-effects, and three-quarters within three years, most women who have ever taken HRT will have no added protection against osteoporosis in their seventies and eighties, when they are most at risk of developing the disease.

That HRT protects against heart disease – the highest cause of death among post-menopausal women – is now questioned by even its most passionate advocates. Far from offering protection against heart attacks and strokes in women who already have heart disease, HRT has been found to increase the risk. Recent studies have shown that in the first year of taking HRT, women have a 52 per cent higher chance of suffering a heart attack. However, HRT may prevent strokes and heart attacks in women who do not already heart disease, although the latest major study to come out of America calls this into question.

As to whether HRT is effective in protecting against Alzheimer's and memory loss, and whether it makes women look and feel younger and sexier, there is no conclusive evidence one way or the other and opinions differ. Women vary in their responses to HRT just as they do to the contraceptive pill and other prescription drugs, and what works for one does not necessarily work for another. Whatever the hype, HRT cannot reverse menopause and keep you young for ever, and for every story of a flagging libido being revived with the help of HRT there's another reporting a severe loss of desire. Other side-effects of HRT include migraines, weight gain, breast tenderness and depression.

More serious are concerns that HRT is linked to an increased risk of blood clots (deep vein thrombosis or DVT), breast cancer, and possibly to other forms of cancer, as well heart disease and strokes. A recent major study in America was halted after it became clear that the brand of HRT used in the trial, a combination of oestrogen and progestin (a form of prosesterone) was damaging rather than improving the health of women taking it. The trial found a 26 per cent increase in invasive breast cancer among the women, who had taken the drug for an average of just over five years, a 41 per cent increase in the risk of strokes, a 22 per cent increase in their risk of heart attacks, and double the risk of blood clots. Another recent trial has found an increased risk of ovarian cancer among women who use oestrogen-only HRT. The risks of taking HRT may not be huge for most women on an individual basis, but for those who are susceptible they are significant.

If you are taking, or thinking of taking, HRT, garner all the information you can and, taking into account your current health and lifestyle (exercise, diet) and your family history, weigh up whether the benefits for you personally outweigh the risks and side-effects. If you decide to stop taking hormones you may wish to do so gradually to minimize the return of menopausal symptoms such as hot flushes and night sweats caused by withdrawal of oestrogen.

Alternative approaches

Concerns about possible links to breast cancer and blood clots are contributing to a backlash against HRT, with women showing a greater interest in natural alternatives such as diet, vitamin and mineral supplements, and herbal cures to help them through their mid-life transition. The herb black cohosh has an oestrogenic effect and has been found to be as effective as HRT in relieving menopausal symptoms, especially in combination with St John's wort. Foods rich in phyto-oestrogens, especially soya and soya-based products like tofu, are claimed to help relieve menopausal symptoms such as hot flushes, night sweats and loss of libido, and many women swear by the effects. Soya is also known to protect against heart disease and may reduce the risk of osteoporosis. Antioxidant vitamins, especially vitamin E, are also important – fruits such as blueberries, strawberries, tomatoes and peppers are highly antioxidant – as are essential fatty acids, found in fish, nuts and seeds, especially linseed (flaxseed).

To provide effective, long-term protection against osteoporosis, heart disease, Alzheimer's and memory loss, combine dietary and other alternative approaches with a healthy lifestyle – keeping active, controlling stress with relaxation and meditation techniques (*see* pages 44–45). For a hormonally healthy start to the day try the following 'smoothie'. A cocktail of antioxidants, plant oestrogens, essential fatty acids, plus calcium for healthy bones, it will boost your energy levels and it tastes great too!

Combine the following ingredients in a blender and liquidize:

1 glass (200 ml) cranberry juice*
30–40 gm soft tofu
1 tablespoon linseed (flaxseed)
1 heaped tablespoon natural yogurt (preferably live,
*   for healthy digestive flora)*
2–3 tablespoons blueberries, fresh or frozen

The consistency will alter according to the kind of tofu you use and the precise amounts – adjust according to taste. Vary by using other kinds of berries and juice, or substituting soya milk for juice. Always use organic or non-genetically modified tofu and soya milk.

* Please note that cranberries, though beneficial in many ways, are naturally bitter and most juices are highly sweetened. If you prefer to avoid sugar, use unsweetened forms of the suggested alternatives.

beauty sleep

Sleep gives our minds and bodies time for rest, recuperation and renewal. The production of growth hormone, which is instrumental in repairing and rebuilding cells, is stimulated during sleep so good-quality, undisturbed sleep is vital to age reversal. Insufficient sleep has an effect on the body similar to that of the ageing process. Besides making us irritable and impairing concentration, sleep deprivation leads to the formation of wrinkles, dark circles under the eyes and general puffiness, and exacerbates age-related disorders such as heart disease and high blood pressure, diabetes and memory loss.

Sleep requirements vary from one individual to another, and as you grow older you tend to need less, but the average adult requirement is about seven or eight hours. If you always feel tired chances are you're not getting enough sleep, and it will show up in haggard looks and a dull complexion. If you have difficulty in getting to sleep (taking longer than 20 minutes) it could well be stress related. If your mind is working overtime, and you cannot switch off work problems, try meditation (*see* pages 121–126) and give yourself time to wind down before bed. Quality of sleep is as important as quantity. If your night is regularly disturbed – this can be due to stress or a variety of other things, not least young children – you may benefit from meditation or other relaxation techniques.

Ways to a good night's sleep

- Create a restful environment in your bedroom. Make it a work-free, television-free zone and clear the clutter.
- Keep your bedroom as quiet and dark as possible, and neither too hot nor too cold – 16–18 degrees centigrade is ideal.
- Keep to regular times of getting up and going to bed, as far as practically possible.
- Ensure you have a comfortable, supportive mattress, and good head support. Your head has the right support when the spinal section in the upper back is level with that of your neck.
- Relax and unwind before going to bed with a book, music, meditation or using the relaxation technique described on pages 115–116.
- Aim to eat your last meal of the day at least two hours before you go to bed.

- Avoid tea, coffee and cola after 6.00 p.m., earlier if you are especially sensitive to caffeine. Take milky drinks and herbal infusions instead.
- Avoid alcoholic nightcaps. Although alcohol can make you drowsy, it interferes with sleep patterns, making you wake in the night, and causes dehydration and headaches.
- Take regular exercise, but not too close to bedtime.
- Relax in a warm bath made fragrant with a few drops of essential oils such as bergamot, geranium, lavender, rose or sandalwood.
- If you wake in the night and cannot get back to sleep, get up and do something relaxing such as reading. Go back to bed when you feel sleepy.

reversing psychological ageing

To the many for whom the spectre of declining mental abilities is of greater concern than fading looks, the good news is that this is by no means inevitable. Even though younger minds may have sharper reflexes, a lifetime of accumulated knowledge, experience and wisdom can give older minds the edge. Mental performance can actually increase into an advanced age so long as you keep active mentally and spiritually. In fact flexing mental muscle is as vital to reversing ageing as physical exercise, and profoundly affects all areas of your life, keeping you young at heart and enriching you emotionally as well as intellectually.

Improving your mind and keeping mentally fit can be as simple as getting a new interest or acquiring new skills. This often involves contact with others and developing your social life, which brings further benefits. The anti-ageing effects of an active sex life within a loving relationship are well known, but many of the same benefits apply to friendships and relationships in which sex plays no part.

Just as the body needs rest and relaxation, so too the mind. One of the brightest stars in the anti-ageing firmament is the practice of meditation. Apart from its spiritual benefits, meditation is a powerful way to relieve stress, the enemy of youth. It also brings mental clarity and helps develop a positive attitude, another quality which plays a huge role in staying young. Optimists live longer, happier lives.

stretch your mind

Some of the clues to keeping the old grey matter in good shape are provided by creative artists, many of whom have lived to a great age and remained highly productive into their seventies and eighties and beyond. Take Picasso and Matisse, who were both working in their eighties, as were the conductor Toscanini, the composer Verdi and the cellist Pablo Cassalls. The contemporary writer Mary Wesley had her first novel published when she was 70 and has written another dozen since. Many artists, like Monet, whose creative genius flowered in his eighties with the painting of his haystack series and the water lilies in his garden at Givenchy, produce their finest work towards the end of their lives. Far from giving in to the constraints of old age, they immerse themselves in creating their art, a complex process involving imagination, memory, attention and intellectual organization. Through the continual exercising of these skills they remain young even at an advanced age.

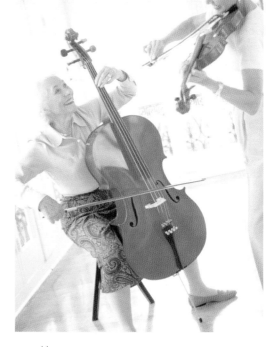

Not everyone can create great art, but we can all cultivate passions and interests – whether golf, playing the piano or learning Chinese – and become absorbed in them. Pursuing new interests stretches your mind, which reverses mental ageing, yet is at the same time relaxing because it takes your mind off problems and anxieties – worry lines are not so-called for nothing. The added bonus is that through acquiring new skills and hobbies you meet new people and broaden your social life – another super-young characteristic, and you become a more interesting person to be around.

a **positive** outlook

Attitude plays a huge role in staying young. People who look on the bright side of life not only live longer, healthier, happier lives, they appear much younger and more energetic than people the same age who focus on problems. Just as success breeds more success, a positive outlook attracts positive things into your life – better jobs with higher remuneration, more stable relationships.

Sadly many people, particularly those with little else in their lives, become increasingly bitter and miserable with age. Like attracts like, and pessimists tend to attract others who enjoy nothing more than a good old moan. Friends fall by the wayside – even the longest-suffering friends and relations can take only so much of a die-hard malcontent. Loneliness becomes a way of life, setting in train a negative spiral of social deprivation, low self-esteem, self-obsession and depression. Fortunately it's a cycle that can be broken, but only with considerable effort.

Get an interest

As just discussed, cultivating interests, especially those you can completely absorb yourself in and that you feel passionate about, takes your mind off niggling anxieties, makes you more interesting (unless your passion is paper clips!) and more fun to be with.

Turn negatives into positives

Take time to become more aware of your thought processes – meditation offers a perfect opportunity for this – and whenever you notice yourself talking or thinking in a negative way make a conscious effort to recast your thoughts in a positive light. Turn losses into opportunities. Accept that although there is much you can do to reverse many aspects of ageing, it is part of the human condition, and the loss of youth heralds the dawning of new wisdom and spiritual insight.

Try using affirmations

Affirmations are strong, positive statements used to change mindset and boost self-esteem through mental repetition. The most famous one, coined by Émile Coué, the pioneer of auto-suggestion, runs: *Every day, in every way, I am getting better and better*. Many people have found affirmations to work for them and help them towards a more optimistic outlook. Affirmations do not have to be mindless platitudes, and should never be unrealistic (as for example a fifty-year-old repeating *I look like a teenager*). Use common sense to create affirmations appropriate to you and your goals, keeping them short, simple, positive and in the present tense, or try *I look and feel young for my age*. Repeat your chosen affirmation(s) like a mantra any time of day.

emotional health

It is often said that true beauty comes from within. Happiness and contentment bestow a radiance which cannot be acquired from even the best of cosmetic treatments. On the other hand anger, fear and other negative emotions leave scars on the face and body. By using positive thinking, meditation and other techniques you can learn to influence and control your emotions. Deep relaxation (*see* page 115) and techniques such as abdominal breathing (*see* page 117) help reduce stress and enable you to take control of strong emotions such as anger, which can lead to unsightly and ageing worry lines.

Develop your social network

Surrounding yourself with people you like is a super-young characteristic and one of the best ways to look and feel great. Research has found that people with a wide circle of friends and social contacts have a lower risk of heart disease and significantly lower blood pressure than those with fewer friends and social contacts. A good network of supportive friends is also excellent for getting you through stressful times, saving you years of stress-related ageing.

Shyness and lack of confidence, which can increase with age, make it hard to initiate new friendships. If you suffer, remember there are millions of people like you who find it difficult to reach out to others. If you possibly can, feel the fear and reach out anyway, accepting that not all people respond to friendly overtures and you may risk rejection. The rewards of making a friendly move are still worthwhile. Your confidence will grow and it will become easier to make and renew friendships.

Of course to keep real friends you need to be a real friend, so be sure to keep your network alive in good times and bad. If you have neglected a friend, make the effort to renew contact. Ten minutes is time enough to drop a quick line, send an email or make a phone call to arrange a date. Expand a diminishing social circle by cultivating new hobbies and interests that involve meeting other people.

Have more sex

A good sex life isn't just enjoyable. Studies show that couples who make love frequently look years younger. This is thought to be because sexual pleasure triggers the release of endorphins – feel-good chemicals – and human growth hormone, both of which slow down the ageing process. Added bonuses are all the emotional and physical benefits a good sexual relationship can bring. The youth-enhancing effects are found only within a committed, loving relationship, however. The benefits are outweighed by the associated risks, anxiety and loss of self-esteem when it comes to casual sex and promiscuous relationships.

spiritual fulfilment

Interest and belief, however free-floating, in a spiritual dimension are consistently associated with better health as well as a longer, more contented life.

It is not that religion in itself is good for you – some people can be damaged by their involvement with religious groups – but rather that the practices associated with religion and spirituality can be highly beneficial. The placebo response demonstrates how beliefs can influence physical health and bring about healing; similarly the power of human belief to change oneself and one's life for the better lies behind techniques such as visualization and positive thinking. Another beneficial aspect of an active spiritual life is that religious and spiritual practices tend to be relaxing. Prayer and meditation, liturgical music, plainsong and chanting, for example, all involve repetition and still the mind, which reduces stress and promotes health and happiness.

The ageing process can be seen as an invitation to delve into the spirit, to discover what, if anything, is eternal and enduring. Meditation is a time-honoured way of opening the doors to the inner realm, even while remaining sceptical about eternal life, and its anti-ageing benefits are exceptional.

• The lotus flower is a symbol of spiritual unfolding.

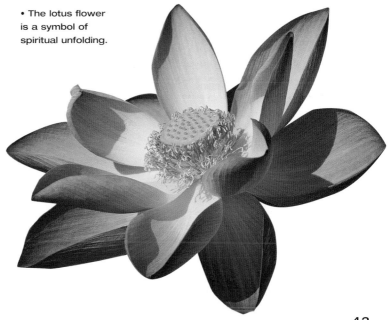

meditation

If you do nothing else to counter the negative aspects of ageing, practising meditation is unbeatable as an all-round anti-ageing therapy. Aside from its spiritual dimension, regular meditation has a profound effect on ageing. Not only is it an effective antidote to stress, one of the main factors contributing to ageing, but meditators have been found to have a biological age many years younger than their chronological age. In tests measuring blood pressure, and visual and auditory performance, short-term meditators were found to have a biological age around five years younger than their real age, and long-term meditators – those who had practised for five years or more – around twelve years.

One of the best kept secrets about meditation is that it also makes you look younger. In fact it is a remarkable beauty treatment. As well as calming your mind, so you emanate an air of inner contentment and serenity, daily meditation is like deep-cleansing your body from the inside out. Your skin is visibly refreshed: lines are smoothed out, bleary eyes and haggard looks replaced by a vibrant glow. This is the real secret of youthful skin and timeless beauty.

As if all these benefits were not enough, meditation sharpens your mind and keeps you young in spirit. The process of meditation is often compared to peeling away the layers of an onion. Layer after layer of habit and conditioning is stripped off, only to reveal more layers underneath. Little by little mental clutter in the form of negative emotions, outworn ideas and prejudices drop away, and you begin to see yourself, your relationships and the world more clearly. Through meditation your senses and intellect are refined, your mind opens and a childlike sense of wonder is restored.

Anyone can meditate. All you need is a place, preferably a quiet one, where you will not be disturbed, and to set aside at least ten minutes. People sometimes worry about the religious connotations of meditation, but it does not involve adopting any beliefs. On the contrary, it can be practised by believers and agnostics alike and is best approached with an open mind.

Perfect posture
This is a classic meditative pose, easier to achieve than the lotus posture, but like the lotus a position of great stability.

Choosing a technique

A variety of meditation techniques, such as using a mantra, visualization and breath-awareness techniques, are described on pages 121–126. Although ways of meditating differ, the techniques share a common purpose: to give your mind something to do, something to focus on. This quietens the constant stream of inner thoughts and mental chatter. When your mind becomes quiet, your consciousness is immersed in the space of peace and stillness within, and you lose yourself in meditation. Meditation techniques are simply doorways into this inner realm. Experiment to find which way is best for you.

The mind is a monkey

One story tells of a seeker who asks a guru to teach him meditation. The guru gives him various instructions, then adds, 'Whatever you do, don't think of a monkey.' Needless to say, the minute the hapless seeker sits to meditate, the image of a monkey leaps into his mind. The more he tries to banish the monkey, the more the monkey takes root in his consciousness.

The story illustrates what happens when you try forcibly to suppress your thoughts. Instead, when you become aware of thoughts, desires and images arising during meditation, adopt a passive attitude towards them, simply noticing them without comment and bringing your attention gently back to your meditation focus.

Sitting for meditation

A still body is conducive to a still mind, so any position you can hold comfortably for at least ten minutes, keeping your spine straight but relaxed, is good. If you can sit in the lotus position (*see* pages 122–123) or the perfect posture (*see* opposite page) without undue discomfort, these are ideal. Otherwise sit in a simple cross-legged position or on a straight-backed chair, with your feet flat on the floor.

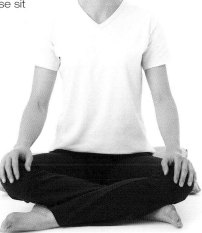

Simple cross-legged position
This is an easy position for most people. As with all meditation positions, the back should be straight but not rigid, and the abdomen relaxed.

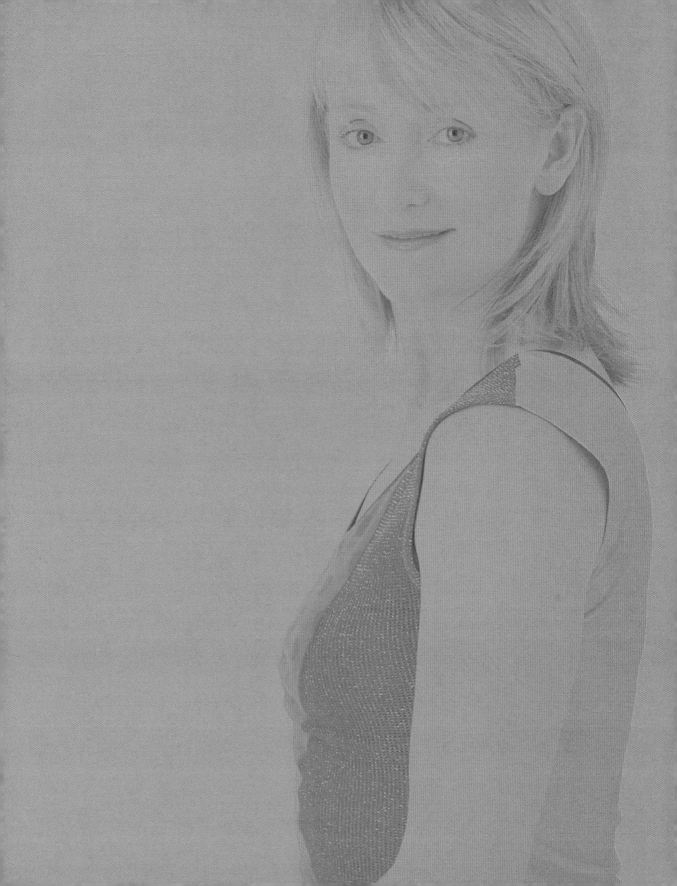

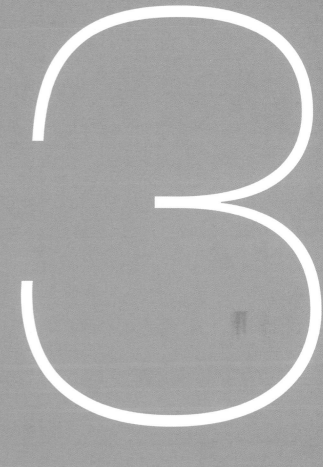

3

ten minute anti-ageing strategies

face & hair

Getting older may be inevitable, but it does not have to mean becoming wrinkled and wizened, or putting up with saggy jowls, dark circles under the eyes, crow's feet and crepey eyelids.

Genes play an important part in determining how your skin ages, but lifestyle plays a much greater role. Prevention is always better than cure, and by protecting your skin from the sun, environmental pollutants and cigarette smoke, as discussed in Part 2, there will be much less damage to repair. Although they can never completely reverse the damage, facial exercises and a good skincare regime can work wonders by improving muscle tone and eradicating fine lines, and giving you a healthy glow. But even the best of anti-ageing creams won't make you look years younger if you are not giving your skin the right nutrients – so be sure to follow a well-balanced diet, such as that outlined on page 20, including enough protein and minimizing sugary and junk foods, and drink eight to ten glasses of water each day.

Greying hair is one of the most noticeable signs of age, but also the most easily hidden. Less obvious is the change in skin tone that comes with age, and if you use colour on your hair, you may need to go a shade or two lighter to balance it. If you have not changed your hairstyle for many years, it may be time to rethink this too. A good cut can take years off your face and the right diet will keep your hair looking healthy and conditioned.

Hitting 40 is a often a trigger for the appearance-conscious – those who are not worried about the possible side-effects or limiting their range of facial expressions – to begin investigating cosmetic procedures such as Botox to suppress and plump out expression lines around the mouth and eyes. Many Botox fans start much younger. The Botoxed 30- or 40-year-old is likely to be considering her (or his) first full face-lift a decade later – cosmetic treatments tend to be addictive. Although they can give an enormous boost to self-esteem, there is always a risk with any kind of drug therapy or surgery, and all cosmetic treatments need to be maintained and repeated. A good face-lift lasts five or six years. Botox and other injectables need to be repeated every four to six months.

Whether or not you wish to resort to surgery, there is an enormous amount you can do to look years – even decades – younger without it, and at the same time save yourself the tens of thousands of pounds it would cost. In fact, if you follow the advice in Part 2, and follow it up with regular ten-minute anti-ageing strategies, you are unlikely to feel the need. And remember that beauty is much more than skin deep, despite the proverb. Inner content gives anyone, of any age, an outer radiance that transcends the most youthful of blooms. Delve into your innermost consciousness and roam around using the meditation techniques on pages 121–126, and your inner beauty will shine out.

daily skin care

Clean skin is healthy skin, and the foundation of any skincare regime is to cleanse properly with a gentle cleanser, day and night, to remove make-up, grime and excess oil, and then hydrate with an appropriate moisturizer for your skin type. Establishing a four-step skincare routine – cleansing, massaging, toning, moisturizing – is the ideal way to ensure you have healthy, clean skin and to slow down or reverse the visible signs of ageing.

Quick cleanse, massage and exfoliation

Facial massage relaxes tense muscles, stretching and releasing them, and gently smoothes away worry lines. It also helps stimulate lymphatic drainage, which reduces puffiness, and increases circulation to the skin, bringing a healthy glow. Incorporate a quick massage into your cleansing routine by applying cleansing cream to your face and neck and then massaging as follows.

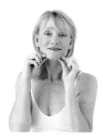

1 Using the flat of your hand, gently but firmly massage from the base of your neck to the jaw line, working your way round from one side of your neck to the other. Alternate your hands in a regular, upward motion, and make at least ten strokes. Then, using the back of your hand, pat the area beneath your chin and along your jaw line quickly and lightly twenty times.

2 Beginning in the centre of your jaw line, make pinching movements with your thumbs and forefingers, working your way up along the jawbone to your ears.

3 Starting at the lower lip, using the pads of your index or middle fingers and applying firm pressure, make stroking movements in a downwards and outward direction, from the lower lip to the chin, then up and out to your earlobes. Continue making a series of ever-decreasing arcs, working your way from the centre of the lower lip to the earlobes, from the outer corners of the mouth to the middle of the ear, base of the nose to the top of the ear, middle of the nose to the temple, inner corner of the eye to the outer. Place your fingers between the brows and sweep them up and out over your forehead, like the rays of the sun, in a series of ever-increasing arcs. (*see* page 52)

4 Finally, still using the pads of the index or middle fingers, trace round the upper and lower ridges of the eye sockets beginning at the bridge of your nose, then sweeping up and round the sockets. Repeat several times, then in a similar way tap gently all round the sockets to stimulate lymph drainage and reduce puffiness around the eye area.

Tissue off or gently exfoliate by rinsing with warm water using a clean, rough-textured flannel. Daily exfoliation speeds up the process of cell turnover and gives you a healthy glow. Use a fresh flannel every day. Tone and moisturize.

Moisturize

There is a bewildering variety of skin creams on the market, many of which make extravagant claims to firm skin, reduce wrinkles and so on. Unfortunately in the real world things are not quite so simple, and one cream will not miraculously make your skin look the way it did twenty years ago. Expensive is not necessarily better, and you certainly do not need to spend a fortune to achieve a healthy, glowing skin.

- **In your twenties** You will need only a light moisturizer. From March until September, use one that includes a sunscreen – SPF 15 – or apply sunscreen on top of your usual moisturizer.

- **In your thirties** You may want to begin using a cream containing fruit acids or alpha hydroxy acids (AHAs), as they are also known, which help repair and brighten up skin by encouraging skin-cell renewal. AHAs are used in many anti-ageing products, but be sure to apply a good sunscreen during the daylight hours if you use them as they can cause greater sensitivity to the damaging ultraviolet rays.

- **In your forties** As you age your skin gets drier, and you may need to adapt your skincare routine and experiment to find a product that suits your particular skin. By your forties you will almost certainly notice a few lines as the collagen is broken down and the skin's elasticity lost, causing the skin to become thinner, and eventually to sag and wrinkle. Boost the skin's collagen production and reduce wrinkles with a retinol-based moisturizer and continue with the sunscreen.

- **In your fifties and beyond** Your skin is likely to be noticeably drier by now as the sebaceous glands become less active, and you may need a richer cream. Active ingredients such as retinol which stimulate collagen and restore radiance are still beneficial, particularly for skin which has had a lot of exposure to the sun. Keep up the sun protection.

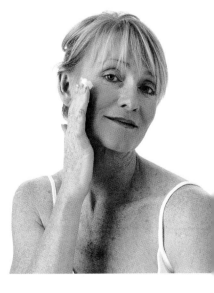

moisturizing facial
massage

Proving the point that expensive is not necessarily more effective, all you need for this excellent anti-ageing treatment, which is best done last thing at night, is a tub of Vaseline or petroleum jelly. Alternatively use any massage oil or face cream of your choice, but Vaseline is an excellent lubricant, which makes it suitable for massaging even the delicate under-eye area, and a highly effective moisturizer.

Cleanse your skin then cover your face with a layer of Vaseline and massage it into your face and neck using light, smooth strokes as described below, but spending two or three minutes on your neck and another two or three minutes on your face.

Now focus on the deep creases and expression lines. Using the pads of your index or middle fingers as before, press firmly into the lines and rock your fingers to and fro across them, at the same time working your fingers along the lines from one end to the other.

Leave the Vaseline on for another three minutes while you relax, then wipe off the excess with a tissue or toner.

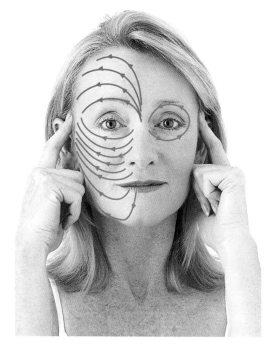

Starting at the lower lip make stroking movements in a downward and outward direction from the lower lip to the chin, then up and out to your earlobes. Continue making a series of ever-decreasing arcs in a similar way up to your eyes.

Now place your fingers between the brows and sweep them up and out over your forehead like the rays of the sun in a series of ever-increasing arcs.

Finally trace around the upper and lower ridges of the eye socket beginning at the bridge of your nose. Repeat several times.

face masks

Face masks are an excellent way to deep cleanse, nourish and smooth skin. DIY buffs like to mix their own: clay or mud (available from chemists) is good for cleansing oily skin, while the flesh of an avocado combined with a teaspoon each of yoghurt and lemon protects against dryness and sun damage and nourishes mature skin. But there is no need to make your own unless you prefer to. There are commercially available masks to suit every type of skin.

Treat yourself once a week, leaving the mask on for ten minutes. For optimum benefits, combine the cleansing effects of your face mask with ten minutes of deep relaxation (*see* page 115).

treat yourself once a week, leaving the mask on for ten minutes

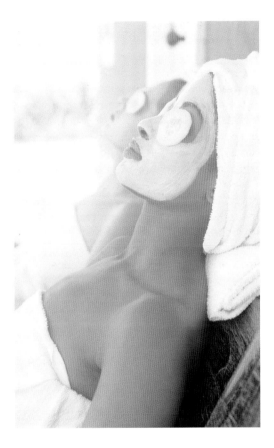

facial exercises

Like the rest of the body, the face has a complex muscular structure which supports the skin and enables facial movement through the contraction and relaxation of muscles. We continually use these muscles to eat, drink and express ourselves. Through minute muscle movements the human face is capable of communicating a huge range of emotions and nuances of feeling with the greatest subtlety: love and tenderness, puzzled amusement, varying degrees of disdain, grief, sadness, anger, indignation and so on. Every time you smile – whether it's an upturned smile of delight or a grim smile of satisfaction – you use as many as 13 different muscles.

Facial exercises build on our unique capacity for facial expression to tone the muscles of the face. Through lack of use facial muscles slacken, and your face begins to lose its youthful contours. Eventually, without the support of firm, toned muscles, skin sags and the whole face develops an ageing droop. As a means to reversing ageing, facial exercise is the polar opposite of Botox, which paralyzes facial muscles where it is injected, reducing the mobility of the face and limiting its expressiveness. Although expression lines form naturally as skin loses its elasticity, facial exercises when done properly do not create wrinkles. By toning the muscles supporting the skin they make you look much younger, yet without any loss of individuality and expression.

In other words, just like the body, the face needs regular workouts – preferably five or six times a week – to keep the muscles toned and firm. All you need is ten minutes a day to give your face a lift, whatever your age. Once you've got the hang of the exercises, which are based on expressions we naturally make, you will find them quick to do, and the beauty is you can do most of them anywhere – in the bath, while you watch television, even in the car, so long as you don't mind what passers-by may think. Pick and mix as appropriate, or do the lot as a complete facial workout. *See also* Eye Exercises (pages 59–60).

Stick out your tongue

For face and neck

Because it involves pulling a particularly grotesque facial expression, not to mention sticking your tongue out, it takes some courage to do this exercise, a classic yoga posture, in public. Known as the lion pose, it strengthens, tones and eases tension in the tongue, jaws, lips, throat and facial muscles. Regular practice tightens the facial muscles, improving appearance, and it is a terrific stress-buster too.

This classic version is done in a kneeling position with hands placed palms down on the knees, but a modified version of the

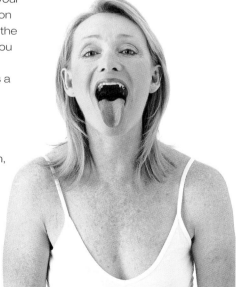

exercise can be done in any comfortable upright position – at your desk or in the driving seat of your car. Take a deep breath then exhale forcefully until your lungs are empty, making an AAARGH sound as you do so. At the same time open your eyes and mouth as wide as possible, stretch your tongue out as far as it will go, as though silently roaring, straighten your arms and stretch out your fingertips, and tense the whole body. Hold the position for as long as you can, then close your mouth and breathe in again through your nose. Relax with a few normal breaths then repeat three or four times.

For neck and throat

Sitting or standing upright, tilt your head back as far as you comfortably can, so you are looking up at the ceiling. Open your mouth and stick your tongue out as far as you can, as if you were trying to touch the ceiling with it. Maintaining the stretch, curl your tongue up as if you were trying to lick the tip of your nose, then back to touch the ceiling, down to lick your chin and back to the starting position. Repeat the movement of the tongue back and forth several times.

Variation

Hold the tongue for five seconds at each of the above positions.

Smile

Thirteen different facial muscles come into play when you smile, which is why simulated smiles form the basis of a wide variety of facial exercises. Try the following exercises to tone up different neck and facial muscle groups and, for an instant lift, do the real thing whenever you can.

For saggy jowls

Sitting or standing upright, pull your bottom lip over the top lip and tilt your chin slightly upwards. Smile, lifting the corners of your mouth towards the top of your ears. You will feel a strong tightening movement in the lower jaw and throat. Hold for five seconds then release. Repeat five times.

For crepey necks and double chins

Begin as for the previous exercise, but instead of holding your smile still, part your lips and begin making a chewing movement while keeping the corners of the mouth pulled back into a smile. After 20 chewing movements release. Repeat two or three times.

55

For neck and cheek muscles

Sitting upright, with your chin level, part your lips slightly and smile
as widely as you can, once a second, directing the outer corners
of your mouth from the jaw line to temples in the following sequence:

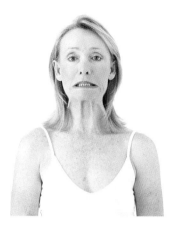 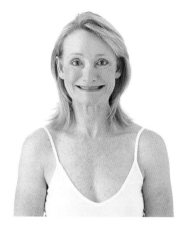 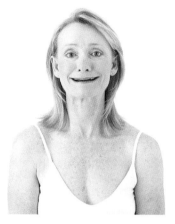

1 The corners of your mouth
curl downwards towards the
jaw line.

2 The corners of your mouth
are pulled outwards towards
the middle of your ear.

3 the corners of your mouth
turn slightly upwards
towards the top of your ear.

4 The corners of your mouth
turn upwards towards your
temples.

5 Repeat the sequence five
or six times.

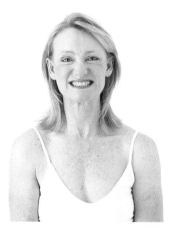

Air-kiss

For chin, cheeks and jaw line

Sitting or standing upright, tilt your head back as far as you comfortably
can, so you are looking up at the ceiling. Purse your lips together and
press them upwards towards the ceiling in an elongated kiss. Hold for
five seconds, trying to reach the ceiling with your lips, then release.
Repeat five times.

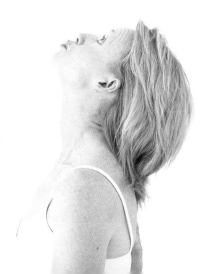

Roll your eyeballs

For upper and lower eyelids

Sit or stand upright with your eyes closed. Keeping the eyelids firmly closed, look upwards, as if you were trying to see something directly above you, then back and downwards to the ground. Repeat ten times.

Raise your eyebrows

For upper eyelids

Sitting or standing upright, close your eyes and raise your eyebrows as high as you can while stretching the lids as much as possible. Hold for five seconds and release. Repeat five times.

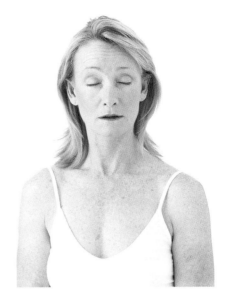

Smooth furrowed brows

To diminish frown lines between the brows

Sit on a chair and rest your elbows on a table in front of you. Lift one hand and place the pads of the thumb and index finger just above the middle of the brows and press them outwards. Close your eyes, relax your face and hold for 30 seconds.

To diminish horizontal frown lines

Sit as above, and place the pads of the fingers of both hands at the top of the forehead along the hairline. Your elbows should be propped up high enough for you to be able to hold your head erect in this position – place books on top of the table beneath your elbows if necessary. Press your fingertips firmly in the direction of the scalp, then close your eyes and relax your face. Hold for 30 seconds.

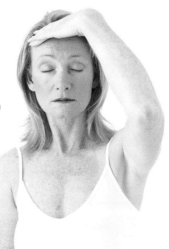
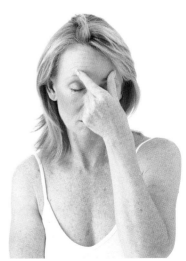

Laugh

A good belly laugh not only keeps you looking young, it keeps you feeling young. Laughter exercises and releases tension not only in the muscles of the face, scalp and neck, but in the torso, shoulders, arms and legs. In fact when you laugh, 16 major organs are affected.

Along with its youth-enhancing benefits, laughter gives you a natural high (it stimulates the production of endorphins), and is a great way to relax and relieve stress. You don't need an endless repertoire of funny jokes or to be brilliantly witty to get laughing. All you need is the ability to see the funny side of life – and stressful situations. As with smiling, if you cannot come up with genuine belly laughter, then fake it till you make it. Laughter – even fake laughter – is infectious.

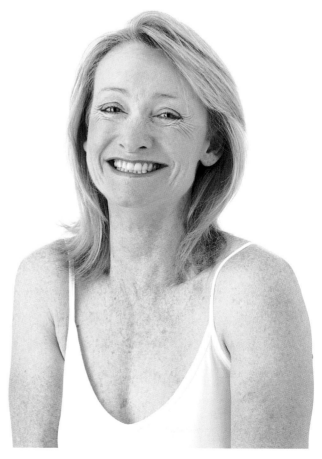

eyes

Eyesight deteriorates with age because the eye muscles no longer work so well and the lens loses its elasticity, causing difficulty in focusing. The most common age-related condition, presbyopia is, along with near sight, noticed by most people in their mid- to late forties when they start finding it difficult to read normal print without reading glasses.

Eye exercises and eye relaxation can help improve vision, especially if regularly practised before much loss of focusing power has occurred. When vision is 20/20 the eyes work easily and need little rest; when vision deteriorates they have to work hard to focus and can quickly become strained and tired, leading to sore eyes, headaches and so on. Palming rests the eyes and releases tension from the muscles, while eye exercises strengthen the muscles and keep the eyes healthy.

Eye exercises

The following exercises strengthen the eyes, relieve eye strain, and can improve vision if practised daily. Follow the eye exercises with palming.

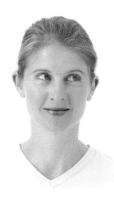

Clock watching

1 Sit with your feet firm and flat on the floor, your back straight, your chest lifted and your shoulders rolling back. Alternatively, if comfortable you can sit on your chair in the lotus or half lotus position (*see* pages 122–123). Rest your hands in your lap or allow them to hang loosely by your sides, and breathe normally throughout the exercise.

2 Imagine a huge clock (the old-fashioned sort with numbers and hands) in front of you a few feet away from your face. Without moving your head, look up to twelve o'clock then down to six o'clock, up to one o'clock then diagonally down to seven o'clock, to two o'clock then across to eight o'clock, and so on round the clock. Repeat each pair of opposites several times before going on to the next pair.

3 Repeat in the opposite direction.

4 Now move your eyes clockwise around the clock, beginning at twelve o'clock, and coming full circle back again. Make slow circles for two or three rounds, then faster for another two or three rounds. Repeat in an anticlockwise direction.

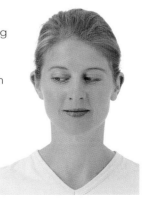

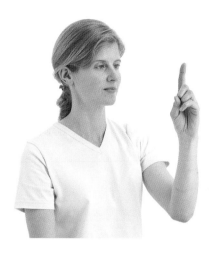

Near-far focusing

1 Sitting as above, hold your forefinger up in front of your nose, about a foot away from you.

2 Focus first on your finger, then on the wall or on any object beyond it (in the middle or far distance). Alternate your gaze to and fro, focusing as clearly as you are able, several times.

Palming

Palm after eye exercises for a few minutes at any time of day to refresh and relax tired eyes.

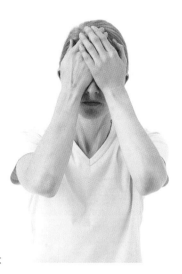

Instructions

1 Sit on a chair with your elbows supported on a table or desk at a height that allows you to cup your hands over your eyes while keeping your back straight. Use books or telephone directories to prop your elbows up if necessary. Alternatively you can sit on the floor with your back supported by a wall, resting your elbows on your knees, or you can lie on the floor on your back with knees raised and feet flat on the floor.

2 Rub your hands together briskly, creating enough friction to warm the palms, then place your cupped hands over your closed eyes without touching them. The outer edges of your palms make firm contact with your face and the fingers are crossed over your forehead, so that all light is excluded.

3 Hold your hands in place for five or ten minutes. Let the heat and dark soothe and relax your eyes.

4 Become aware of your breathing. Feel your eyes becoming energized and invigorated as you breathe in, feel them relaxing as you breathe out tension.

Glasses and sunglasses

Wearing sunglasses helps prevent wrinkles forming around the eyes by stopping you squinting in bright sunlight and, more important, protecting the delicate skin around the eye area from harmful ultraviolet rays. Wear UV-protective glasses whenever you are in the sun, and goggles when swimming. And remember out of date frames can be ageing. Change them every couple of years.

tooth care

After eyes, the mouth is the most noticeable facial feature, and a gleaming set of white teeth the prerequisite of a young and dazzling smile. Ageing combined with poor oral hygiene can, however, play havoc with your teeth and mar the most perfect of smiles. One of the main effects of dental ageing is tooth discolouration and staining, the worst offenders being nicotine, tea and coffee. The good news is that stains can be effectively removed with whitening products available from chemists or, for more stubborn stains, professional tooth whitening. Dental technology has advanced so far that aesthetic dentists can do almost anything, for a price, from realigning teeth to changing their colour, shape and size. But not even the best cosmetic dentistry can fix teeth that have fallen out or gums that have receded.

If you don't want to appear long in the tooth, a sign of receding gums, and you'd rather avoid dentures, another serious sign of age caused by tooth decay, then go back to basics and invest in a good toothbrush (many dentists recommend electric toothbrushes which give the gums a good massage), fluoride toothpaste and some dental floss. Correct brushing and flossing keeps teeth clean, bright and healthy, and prevents the build-up of plaque, which causes dental decay and gum disease. Brush thoroughly for at least two minutes twice a day and change your toothbrush every month, or more often if the bristles have splayed out (a sign that you may be brushing incorrectly). If you are unsure how to brush your teeth correctly ask your dentist or oral hygienist to demonstrate. At least once a day, as an adjunct to brushing, gently floss your teeth to remove plaque and food particles caught in the gaps between them and around the gums.

As well as regular brushing and flossing, for gleaming teeth that last a lifetime avoid smoking and follow a healthy diet which minimizes sugary foods. And don't forget your six-monthly dental check-ups – damage caught early is much easier to repair.

hair and scalp

If you feel good about your hair you're likely to feel good about life. A shining, lustrous mane of hair is rightly considered one's crowning glory, and mid-life hair loss and thinning, along with greying, can really erode self-confidence.

Grey hair is one of the features most associated with age, but one of the easiest to remedy. If your hair is beginning to grey and you want to colour it at home, try going a shade or two lighter than your natural colour. As your hair loses pigment, so does your skin tone, and strong colour can look hard. Lighter colour will give the illusion of highlights and result in a softer, more youthful look.

Just as ageing skin can lose its radiance, hair tends to lose its natural sheen as you age. Greying hair in particular changes its texture, and looks less glossy. Counter this with weekly conditioning treatments such as the ten-minute conditioning head massage described on the opposite page. Following a good diet with plenty of protein, fresh fruit and vegetables, such as the one described on pages 20–21, will also help keep hair healthy and shiny.

More difficult to deal with is the hormonally related loss of hair that affects many men and a significant number of post-menopausal women. Nevertheless there is a lot you can do to improve the situation. Male-pattern baldness – which also affects a few women – is hereditary, but hair growth can be improved with prescription medicines, especially when complemented by dietary and lifestyle changes where appropriate (see Part 2). Hormonal changes at mid-life cause some degree of hair thinning in almost 40 per cent of women. Chronic stress is also a cause, as it reduces circulation to the scalp and deprives it of the nutrients that stimulate hair growth.

To avoid bad-hair days, make the most of what you've got by:

• getting a good haircut – a good cut can take years off your face.
• using gentle shampoo and not washing your hair more than two or three times a week. Use conditioner on the ends only.
• using a comb rather than a brush on wet hair, which can easily be stretched and damaged. Begin combing the ends of the hair and work up.
• maximizing volume by bending your head down as you blow-dry it. Experiment with professional products designed to give extra volume.
• massaging your scalp regularly. Once a week combine this with oil or intensive hair conditioner and leave on for five or ten minutes before shampooing.

Ten-minute hair conditioning head massage

Coconut oil, much used in the manufacture of hair products and cosmetics, is the traditional choice for head massage. It is extremely light, which makes it excellent not only for massaging and conditioning the hair and scalp, but for protecting the skin all over the body. Olive or almond oil make good substitutes. If using coconut oil – available in health food and Asian stores – you may prefer to warm it a little beforehand as it is solid at room temperature. Otherwise scoop it up with your fingers – your body heat will liquefy it in a matter of moments. If using liquid oil, apply with cotton wool along partings spaced out regularly over your scalp.

Massage for a few minutes as described below – you may find it helpful to bend your head forward – then stroke your fingers through your hair to ensure the oil reaches the ends. Leave on for five or ten minutes, or best of all overnight, before washing off.

Scalp massage

Cultures like that of India, which put a premium on long luxuriant hair, have a tradition of head massage which is thought to improve the health and condition of the hair and make it grow thicker. Although not a cure for baldness, scalp massage stimulates the circulation of blood to the area and relaxes any tightness of the scalp caused by stress, which helps promote hair growth. Best of all, it feels fantastic – especially if someone else does it for you.

You can massage your hair dry or wet, using shampoo, conditioner, oil or nothing at all. There is no 'right' way to massage, but aim to move the scalp with the fingers, rather than the fingers over the scalp, using the pads of your fingertips in small circular movements with a comfortable degree of pressure. To ensure you work over the entire scalp, spread your fingers and work methodically from the top of your scalp to the sides, and from the front of your head to the base of your neck.

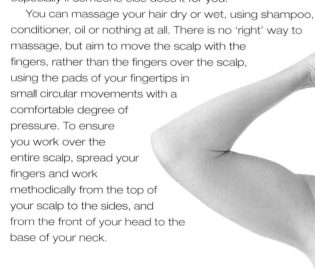

body

The hallmarks of a youthful body are good posture, correct weight, toned muscles, suppleness, strength and a spring in the step. These qualities are achieved and maintained through good nutrition (*see* pages 20–21), regular exercise and good posture.

Good posture, whether sitting, standing or moving, is probably the quickest way to knock ten years – and ten pounds – off your appearance. Work on it with the body check (*see* pages 66–69) or with any of the other exercises in this book which are based on yoga and Pilates, both of which help realign your body.

Exercise needs vary, but you should aim for at least an hour and a half of exercise each week, and ideally twice this much, exercising at least five days a week. This can be taken in ten-minute slots and should include aerobic (for the cardiovascular system, i.e. heart and blood vessels), weight-bearing and weight-resistance (strengthening, good for bones) and stretching (for suppleness and flexibility) exercise. Combining all of these are the sun salutations (*see* pages 72–73), a wonderful sequence for all-round fitness. Target specific areas, especially those prone to the effects of gravity, with the gravity-defying exercises (*see* pages 82–107) designed especially for the purpose. Yoga is well known for reversing the effects of ageing, and inverted postures such as the headstand and shoulderstand (*see* pages 74–81) are particularly prized for their rejuvenating effects.

If you are over 40 and/or unfit, start any programme of exercise gently. One of the simplest and most natural ways to get fit is by taking regular, brisk, ten-minute walks – preferably two or three times a day. Beware ware of overdoing it, however. Like crash dieting, obsessive exercising rarely achieves its goals. If you overdo it you will feel worse, not better, and not keep it up. That said, you will need to push yourself slightly beyond your comfort zone to increase your fitness. The exercise routines in the following pages are not beyond the capabilities of most people, though to begin with you may work slowly and do few, if any, repeats. Time and familiarity with the routines will speed up the process and you will be able to accomplish more. The good news is that the less fit you are, the more and the quicker you will notice the benefits of exercise. Others will too!

Finally, don't forget to look after your skin and feet. Skin becomes drier with age, so if you suffer from dry, rough skin or dry, cracked heels, turn to pages 110–111 to restore your skin's radiance.

the **body** check

Correcting poor posture takes years off your appearance in an instant, making you look leaner, slimmer, more confident and relaxed. Good posture elongates the spine and ensures that your body weight is evenly spread around your centre of gravity in the lower spine and pelvis. As well as dramatically improving appearance, maintaining good posture protects against and combats a wide range of age-related health problems.

Poor posture, by contrast, is not only ageing but leads to a whole host of health problems. Habitual stooping and slouching puts your joints out of alignment and distributes your body weight unevenly, causing continual physical stresses and strains. The end result is stiffness, aches and pains, especially back pain; acceleration of the degenerative effects of the ageing process on the spine and the rate of loss of bone density, leading to fractures and the classic 'dowager's hump'; a reduction of lung capacity; impaired digestion; exhaustion, lethargy and much more.

good posture takes years off your appearance making you look slimmer and more confident

A sedentary lifestyle – days spent hunched up over a desk and evenings slumped on a sofa watching television – exacerbates poor postural habits, as hunched shoulders tend to stay that way when you get up and shuffle off for a coffee. If your posture is less than perfect, work on it with the body check, a quick way to tune into your body, correct poor posture, release tension and relax. You can do it anywhere – queuing up at the supermarket checkout, birdwatching or at your desk. Use the sitting and standing versions as appropriate, and carry the principles of good posture into walking and all other physical activities.

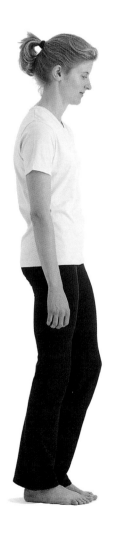

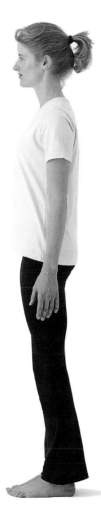

Body check: standing

Instructions

1 Standing wherever you happen to be, bring your attention to your body and scan it from the tips of your toes to the top of your head, noting where there is any tension or imbalance.

2 Rest your arms at your sides, allowing your hands to hang loosely, palms facing your thighs. Bring your feet together so your weight is evenly distributed over the inner and outer sides of the feet, but without dropping the arches and inner ankles.

3 Bring your shoulders back and down, gently stretching and elongating your spine and the back of your neck. Hold your chin level and tuck in your pelvis (imagine that you had a tail and you were trying to tuck it down between your legs).

4 Breathing slowly and evenly, adjust the posture, continuing to lengthen upwards. Imagine a golden thread running from the base of your spine to the crown of your head, gently lifting you up. Your weight should now be centred over your pelvis, with your head comfortably balanced above your neck so that head, neck, spine, pelvis, legs and feet are in a straight, but relaxed line.

5 Relax your face. Allow your lips to part slightly and rest your tongue in the base of your mouth. Soften your jaw and your throat. Soften your gaze and smile inwardly.

6 Mentally scan your body again, noting any tension spots. Where you find tension, breathe into it. Breathe in energy, breathe out tension.

Focus points

- Check your shoulders are even and your hips level and directly beneath your shoulders.
- Your head should be in neutral position, not tilted to one side, and the chin straight.
- If anything there should be more weight on your heels than your soles.

Body check: sitting

Good sitting posture centres your body weight evenly over your sitting bones and ensures that the pelvis is in neutral position, neither tilting forward so your back is overarched, nor backwards so you slump. Developing good sitting posture is particularly important if you spend long hours working at a desk as it reduces the likelihood of back pain and keeps your chest open so you breathe more efficiently and have more energy.

Instructions

1 Sit on a chair with a firm base, such as an office or dining chair, with your feet firm and flat on the floor (place books or telephone directories beneath them if necessary), hip-width apart, knees directly above them and slightly lower than your hips. Alternatively sit on the floor in any of the cross-legged positions suggested for meditation (*see* pages 44–45 and 122–123). Rest your hands in your lap or allow them to hang loosely by your sides.

2 Breathe in deeply, feeling your abdomen swell, your side ribs expand and the top of your chest lift. Lengthen your spine and extend the back of your neck without tensing the muscles, so you are sitting comfortably erect. Keep your chin tucked in.

3 Breathing out, lower your shoulders and draw them back gently, pressing your shoulder blades into your back.

4 Take one or two more deep breaths, stretching and elongating your spine upwards with each inhalation, keeping your shoulders down and back and your chin tucked in. The weight of your upper body should now be centred over your sitting bones, your abdomen back and up. Imagine a golden thread in the centre of your spine extending from the base vertically upwards through the crown of your head, gently drawing you up.

5 Hold the posture and, breathing naturally, consciously relax your whole body, being sure to soften and relax your face, jaw and tongue, which hold a lot of tension.

6 Mentally scan your body from the tips of your toes to the crown of your head, noting any tension spots. Where there is tension in your body, visualize yourself breathing into it. Breathe in relaxation, breathe out tension.

7 Maintain the position for ten minutes.

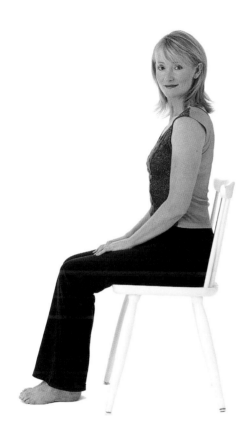

a good sitting posture is very important if you spend long hours at a desk

Focus points

- Check your shoulders are even and your hips directly beneath them.
- Your head should be in neutral position, not tilted to one side, and the chin straight.
- Closing your eyes will help you focus inwards.

Your body should now feel poised, relaxed and centred. If you find sitting this way a strain it is probably due to weak back muscles, resulting from poor posture. Through regular practice they will strengthen and sitting well will become habitual.

walking workouts

Walking is our natural way of moving, and one of the quickest and most effective ways to overall fitness, depending on how often and how fast you walk. The beauty of walking is that it can be done anywhere – though for both mental and physical health a scenic route is preferable to walking on busy, polluted roads, is suitable for people of all ages, and has been shown to reverse ageing, even in the elderly. One study found that a walking programme for people in their seventies reversed more than 20 years of declining lung capacity, while another found that elderly people who walk several times a week decrease their risk of hip fractures and disability, and improve their ability to climb stairs, bend, crouch and kneel.

Benefits

Because it is low-impact, walking has less potential than jogging or running for injury to the knees and other joints, yet regular, brisk walking offers all the same benefits, including:

- strengthening of the cardiovascular system, lowering blood pressure and cutting your risk of heart disease and strokes
- improving circulation and bringing a healthy glow to your skin
- improving lung capacity and promoting an increased supply of oxygen to the body
- strengthening bones and muscles, and reducing the risk of osteoporosis and fractures
- promoting spinal health and reducing back pain by helping to keep the spinal discs lubricated
- encouraging weight loss in the overweight
- improving endurance and increasing energy levels
- reducing stress and promoting emotional and spiritual well-being

Walk tall

The way you walk can reveal a lot about your age! A youthful walk is based on the principles of good posture (*see* page 66–67), maintaining a straight but not rigid back, head poised and looking neither up nor down, shoulders even and relaxed, pelvis tucked in, weight centred over your heels. Take long, even, flowing strides, smoothly transferring your weight from one foot to the other. Keeping up as brisk a pace as you comfortably can will bring the most rapid results in terms of getting fit and reversing ageing.

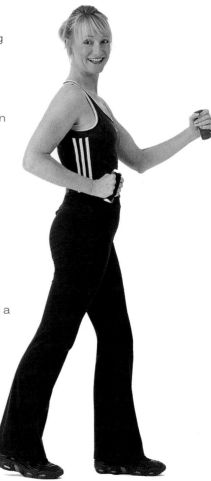

Healthy feet

Our feet are designed for walking, which exercises and strengthens their muscular structure. However, it is important to wear the right shoes or trainers, particularly if you want to alternate between walking and jogging or running. Choose good-quality, comfortable shoes that provide adequate cushioning and support, while allowing your feet to breathe and your toes room to move.

If you wear high heels most of the time it is a good idea to warm up and stretch your calf muscles before a brisk walk, and essential if you are combining walking with running. The Achilles tendon tends to shorten if you wear heels and can be easily injured if abruptly stretched by high-impact exercise such as running.

Combined walking and jogging/running workout

It has been suggested by an eminent plastic surgeon that, apart from sun damage and smoking, running is the main cause of premature skin ageing and wrinkles. This is because the facial skin is pulled away from the muscles supporting it, bobbing up and down with the impact of each pace. However other experts disagree and, being high-impact, running is one of the best bone-strengthening activities. So if you want to build up fitness with more vigorous exercise than walking alone, alternate with jogging or running. Be sure to stretch your calf muscles beforehand to prevent injury to the knees and Achilles tendons, and wear good-quality running shoes or trainers which will provide adequate support.

Calf stretch

Stand facing a wall with your left leg about one to one and a half feet away from it, and your right leg three to three and a half feet away, keeping both feet flat on the floor. Keeping your back leg straight while gently bending your front knee, place your palms with fingers upward on the wall at shoulder level, shoulder width apart, so your arms are straight. Press against the wall for a minute or two, feeling the stretch in the back of the left leg all the way from the Achilles tendon through the calf to the back of the knee. Swap the position of the legs and repeat.

sun salutations

The current popularity of flowing and fast-paced styles of yoga such as ashtanga has ensured that the sequence of movements known as the sun salutations has become a core practice for many Westerners, and with good reason. A condensed yoga programme in itself, the sequence oxygenates the blood and energizes the whole system, bringing increased suppleness to the spine, building strength and stamina, and toning the entire body.

Performed fairly rapidly on rising sun salutations provide an invigorating start to the day, bringing a healthy glow and youthful colour to the cheeks. Performed slowly, they relieve physical tension and make a great way to relax and unwind.

There are many variations of the sun salutations. The version described here is the one most often found in yogic literature, and one of the easiest to learn.

Position 1: Mountain, hands in prayer position Stand upright with your feet together, weight evenly spread over the soles of your feet, then bring your palms together in front of your chest in the prayer position. Breathe out.

Position 2: Hands up Breathing in, stretch your arms up and slightly back, palms facing forward.

Position 3: Head to knees Breathing out, bend forwards from the hips, placing your palms flat on the floor beside your feet and bringing your face as close to your knees as you can. You may need to bend your knees in this position to begin with.

Position 4: Lunge Without moving your hands or left foot, breathe in and stretch back with your right leg, placing the knee on the floor and curling the toes under. Your left knee should then be above your left ankle. Arch your back and look up.

Position 5: Plank Holding your breath, bring your left leg back alongside the right, supporting your body on your hands and toes. Head, back, legs and heels should all be in a straight line.

Position 6: Eight parts position Breathing out, bend your arms and lower knees, chest and forehead to the floor, keeping the elbows high and hands firmly down.

Position 7: Cobra Breathing in, lower your hips to the floor and slide forward so your toes point back. Straighten your arms, lift your chest and take your head back.

Position 8: Downward-facing dog Breathing out, curl your toes under and lift your hips up into an upside-down V shape. Push back on your heels, trying to place your feet flat on the floor. Drop your head in between your arms.

Position 9: Lunge Breathing in, bring your right leg forward between your hands and at the same time lower your left knee to the floor. Arch your back and look up. This is the mirror image of position 4.

Position 10: Head to knees Breathing out, bring the left leg in line with the right, and assume position 3 again.

Position 11: Arms up Breathing in, extend your arms up and back, repeating position 2.

Position 12: Mountain Breathing out, lower your arms to your sides or, if you are performing another round, resume the starting position.

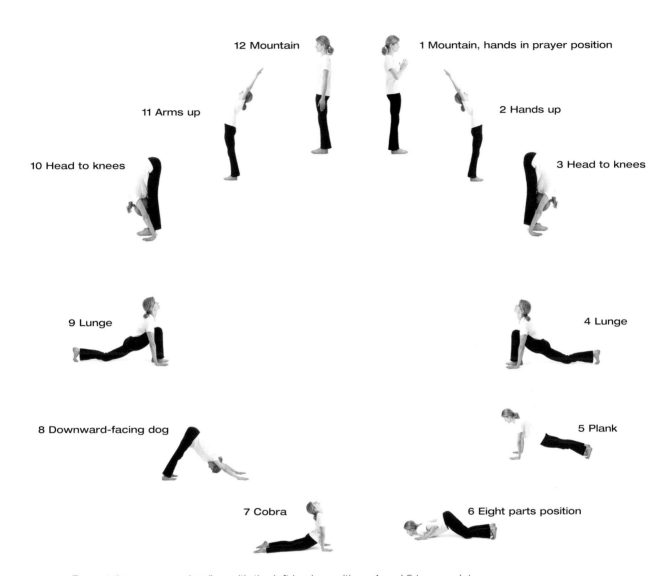

12 Mountain

1 Mountain, hands in prayer position

11 Arms up

2 Hands up

10 Head to knees

3 Head to knees

9 Lunge

4 Lunge

8 Downward-facing dog

5 Plank

7 Cobra

6 Eight parts position

Repeat the sequence leading with the left leg in positions 4 and 9 to complete one full round of sun salutations. Begin with one round, practising the sequence slowly and carefully, perfecting each posture and moving as smoothly as you can from one position to the next, gradually adding a round a day until you have built up to 12 rounds. After completing the sun salutations lie down and relax for a few minutes in the corpse position (*see* page 115). To complement the sun salutations do the half moon pose on page 87, which will give the spine a lateral stretch and tone the waist and abdomen.

headstands and shoulderstands

'You are old, Father William,' the young man said,
'And your hair has become very white;
And yet you incessantly stand on your head –
Do you think, at your age, it is right?'
LEWIS CARROLL

Father William was on to something, for among all the postures of hatha yoga, a system well known for its anti-ageing effects, the inverted positions, in which the head is lower than the rest of the body, are considered the most rejuvenating of them all. When you are upside down the pull of gravity is reversed, increasing the circulation of blood to the neck, face and brain. Daily practice of inverted positions – the headstand and/or the shoulderstand – for five or ten minutes is said to aid concentration, increase intellectual power, boost memory and improve looks.

Other parts of the body also benefit, including internal organs such as the lungs and the heart, which effectively gets a holiday in these positions. The spinal column is strengthened, and performing the shoulderstand variations will increase its flexibility. Among the many other benefits claimed are relief from stress, insomnia, constipation, and menstrual and menopausal problems. Inverted postures also improve the appearance of the body, countering sagginess around the abdomen and, by giving the leg veins a rest, prevent and relieve varicose veins.

If you cannot manage the headstand, or find it a strain, do the milder shoulderstand, which brings similar benefits. If you practise both, always do the headstand first. Wait a couple of hours after eating, three after a heavy meal, before going into inverted positions.

Headstand

Known as the king of the yoga postures, the headstand involves balancing the weight of the body on the elbows, forearms and hands, which are interlocked to form a firm triangular base. Your weight should be evenly distributed between the arms and the head.

The headstand is an exhilarating and rejuvenating posture, but should be avoided if you are pregnant or menstruating, if you have high blood pressure, heart problems, brittle bones which could easily be broken, ear or eye disorders such as glaucoma or a detached retina, or are suffering from any injury, especially to the neck. If you are overweight, elderly or unfit, do not attempt the headstand until you can stay comfortably in the shoulderstand for three to five minutes.

Instructions

1 Kneel on the floor, with a folded blanket in front of you, and place your forearms on the blanket, clasping each elbow with the opposite hand.

2 Without moving your elbows, release the hands and clasp them together, interlacing your fingers, to form a secure base in the form of a tripod. The distance between your elbows should not be more than the width of your shoulders.

3 Place the crown of your head on the blanket, so that the back of your head is firmly pressed against the palms of your hands.

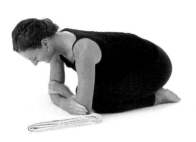

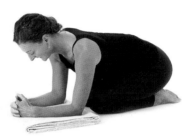

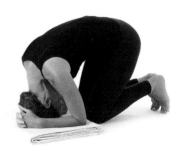

4 Straighten the knees so your body forms an upside-down V, then walk your feet in towards your head as far as you can, making sure that you are lifting your shoulders.

5 Bend the knees and raise the legs upwards until the body is erect and the legs vertical.

6 Hold for just a few seconds to begin with, gradually increasing to five or ten minutes.

7 Come down gently and slowly, and rest back in the child's pose, kneeling with your forehead onthe floor or blanket and your arms, palms upward, on either side of the body.

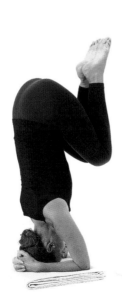

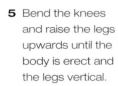

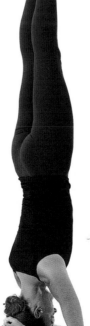

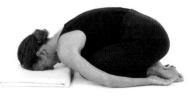

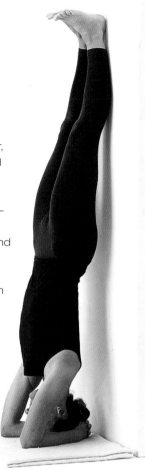

Focus points

- Beginners should practise against a wall or, better still, a corner, placing their interlaced hands two or three inches away from the wall.
- Ensure you place the crown of your head – the very top of it, on which you could balance a book if you were standing up, and not the part nearer your forehead – on the blanket, so your chin is tucked in. Coming up with your chin out will place pressure on the neck and cause incorrect alignment of the spine.
- Keep the tailbone in so the spine is erect, not arched.
- Try to lift your shoulders away from the floor by pressing the forearms down.

Shoulderstand

If the headstand is the king of yoga positions, the shoulderstand is the queen and, like the headstand, it is a relaxing and rejuvenating pose, offering similar benefits. In this position the weight of your body is supported by your shoulders and blood circulation increases in the neck, with a beneficial effect on the thyroid and parathyroid glands. Holding the posture increases spinal strength and flexibility, and firms and tones the entire body. The shoulderstand is also highly recommended for people who want to lose weight as it compresses the thyroid gland and balances the metabolic rate.

The shoulderstand is suitable for most people, but should be avoided during menstruation. If you have high blood pressure go into the plough position (*see* page 79) for two or three minutes first, and do not stay in the posture if you feel pressure in the neck or head.

Ten minutes in the shoulderstand and its variations brings maximum benefits and acts as a powerful restorative. If you practise both the shoulderstand and the headstand, always do the headstand beforehand. Follow the shoulderstand with the fish position.

Instructions

1 Place one or more thick blankets on the floor and lie down with your back and shoulders on the blanket and your head resting on the floor, chin tucked in towards your chest. Bring your arms to your sides, palms downwards, and press the shoulders down. Bend your knees and place your feet flat on the floor close to your buttocks.

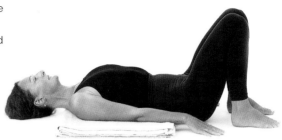

2 On an inhalation slowly and smoothly lift your legs, hips and trunk up vertically, bending your elbows to support your back with your palms, and pressing your elbows firmly into the blanket. Using your hands to lift your upper back, straighten your back as much as possible and stretch your legs vertically upwards, keeping your tailbone in.

3 Hold for half a minute to begin with, building up to ten minutes, including the plough and fish positions and any variations.

4 To come out of the position lower your legs over your head and roll your back down along the blanket slowly and smoothly, keeping your head on the floor.

Focus points

- If you have difficulty getting into the position, begin by lying close to a wall and lift your hips up by pressing your feet into the wall.
- Coming into the plough position (*see* page 79) for a minute before holding the shoulderstand can improve the latter by helping you to extend the body upwards.
- Bring your elbows as close together as you can, and your hands as close to the shoulders as possible. The closer they are, the more you will be able to raise your body.

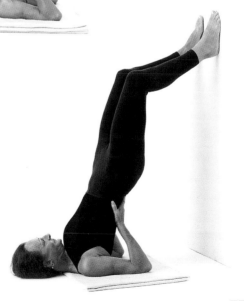

Variations

Once you can comfortably hold the shoulderstand for a few minutes a range of variations can be performed bringing increased strength and flexibility to the spine and enabling you to hold the position for longer. Many of the variations can also be performed in the headstand.

Variation 1 Bending your knees sideways, press the soles of your feet together. Hold for 30 seconds then come back into shoulderstand.

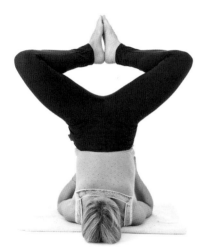

Variation 2 Spread your legs as wide as you can. Hold for 30 seconds then come back into shoulderstand.

Variation 3 Keeping your left leg upright, lower the right leg horizontally over your head. Hold for 30 seconds then come back into shoulderstand. Repeat reversing the legs.

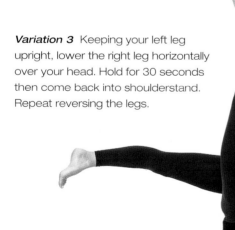

Variation 4 As variation 3, but this time lower each leg to the floor, curling your toes inwards towards your head.

Variation 5 Bending your hips slightly forward, fold your legs into the lotus position (*see* page 122) then extend your trunk and knees upwards. Hold for as long as comfortable then come back into shoulderstand and repeat, crossing your legs in reverse fashion.

Variation 6 As variation 5, but this time lowering the knees over your head.

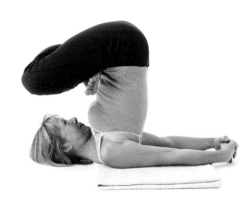

Plough

This posture offers the same benefits as the shoulderstand, and stretches the back of the body. Like shoulderstand variation 6 above, the plough position elongates the entire spine, keeping it supple and youthful, and relieving backaches. Regular practice also stimulates digestion and slims the abdomen, hips and legs.

Instructions

1 Come into shoulderstand, using a folded blanket under your shoulders as before.
2 On an exhalation, keeping the legs straight, lower them over your head, bending from the hip, to rest your toes on the floor, curling them under.
3 Stretch your arms behind your back and clasp the hands together, interlacing the fingers.
4 Hold for as long as you comfortably can, then unroll slowly, keeping your legs straight. When your buttocks touch the floor slowly lower the legs.

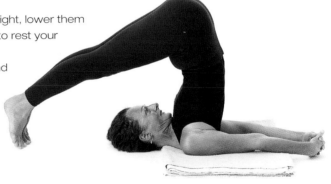

Focus points

- Try to keep your legs straight as you come down into plough, but bend your knees if this is too hard on your back. Once your feet touch the floor or your support (*see* the focus point below), straighten the legs.
- If you cannot comfortably touch the floor with your legs straight, rest your toes on a strategically placed chair or against a wall.
- To avoid straining the back, bend from the hips to come into the plough.

Variations

Once you can comfortably hold the plough position, practise any of the following variations.

Variation 1 From plough position extend your arms behind your head and grasp the toes, resting the backs of the hands on the floor.

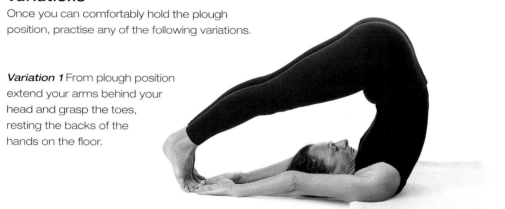

Variation 2 From plough position spread the legs as wide as you can, then stretch your arms out behind your head to grasp the toes, keeping your back lifted.

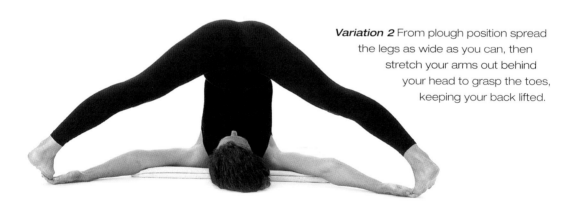

Variation 3 From plough position bend your knees and bring them down to rest on the floor or as near to the floor as you can, either side of your ears. Take your arms behind your knees, clasping the opposite arm with each hand.

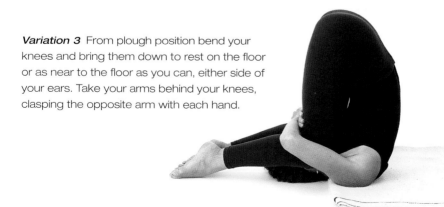

Fish

This position is an excellent couter-pose to the shoulderstand and plough positions, relieving any strain in the neck and back. The spine is strengthened and any tendency to round shoulders corrected. The classic version of this yoga posture is done in the lotus position, but only attempt it if you can sit in the lotus comfortably for at least five minutes.

Instructions (easier version)

1 Lying flat on your back with your legs extended and your feet together, bring your arms under your buttocks, palms face down.
2 Bend your elbows and press them into the floor, using them to raise your chest.
3 Arching your back as much as you can, let your head drop back, placing the crown of your head on the floor.

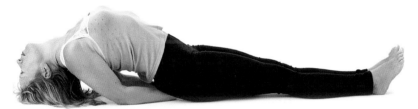

4 Hold for half as long as the shoulderstand, including variations, or for as long as you can keeping the chest lifted.

Instructions (classic version)

1 Sit in the lotus position (*see* page 122).
2 Leaning back, place your elbows on the floor.
3 Arching your back as much as you can, place the crown of your head on the floor.
4 Catch hold of your toes.
5 Hold for half as long as the shoulderstand.

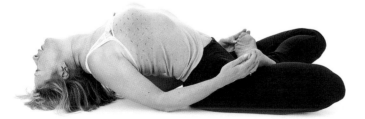

Focus points

- Keep your knees to the ground.

gravity-defying exercises

The exercises on the following pages are designed to lift and tone those parts of the body which are particularly prone to the effects of gravity – and ageing. Try them individually to become familiar with the movements, then mix as appropriate or try the suggested sequences on page 106–107.

Deep abdominal toning

These exercises improve your shape by strengthening the deep abdominal muscles and increasing core strength. This in turn helps support the lower back and guards against and alleviates lower-back pain. The exercises also lower the risk of incontinence in women by activating the pelvic floor. This action is increased if you contract and release the muscles around the vagina as you exhale. Correct breathing is a vital component of success.

Abdominal breathing

Follow these breathing instructions where indicated.

Instructions

1 Lie on your back with your knees bent and feet flat on the floor hip-distance apart.
2 Place your hands on your lower abdomen in between your pubis and your navel.
3 Breathing through your nose, begin to lengthen your exhalations and think of directing them into the lower abdomen. You should feel the downward movement of the abdomen towards the lower back with your hands.
4 During the inhalations try to maintain the depression of the lower abdomen.
5 Take six directed breaths, taking a normal breath in between if you experience any discomfort.

Focus points

- You are not trying to suck the abdomen down to the floor as you exhale. However, you should feel a tension deep in the pelvic floor.
- If you feel any pressure in your head, you are trying too hard.

Pelvic tilts

This is a continuation of the abdominal breathing exercise described above.

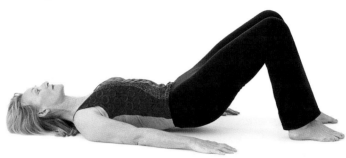

Instructions

1 Place your hands palms down on the floor by your sides.
2 Breathing as above, on an exhalation curl your pelvis away from the floor into your naval.
3 Maintain the pelvic tilt during the next inhalation and exhalation, and roll down on the following inhalation.
4 Repeat six times.

Focus point

- Keep the back of your waist on the floor.

Elbow lift

Instructions

1 Start on your elbows and knees, with your hands together so that your elbows are in front of your shoulders, your knees behind your hips, with your toes tucked under as shown in the illustration. Keep your head level.

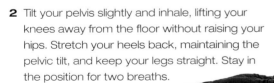

2 Tilt your pelvis slightly and inhale, lifting your knees away from the floor without raising your hips. Stretch your heels back, maintaining the pelvic tilt, and keep your legs straight. Stay in the position for two breaths.
3 Repeat three to six times.

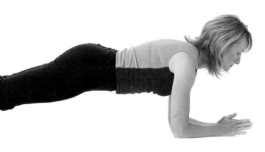

Focus points

- If you cannot keep your hips down, go back to the initial position and move your knees farther back.
- Press your elbows into the floor and take your shoulders away from your ears.

Leg lowering

Follow the abdominal breathing throughout this exercise.

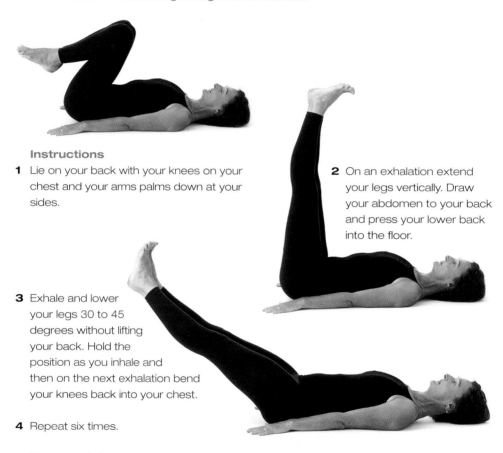

Instructions

1 Lie on your back with your knees on your chest and your arms palms down at your sides.

2 On an exhalation extend your legs vertically. Draw your abdomen to your back and press your lower back into the floor.

3 Exhale and lower your legs 30 to 45 degrees without lifting your back. Hold the position as you inhale and then on the next exhalation bend your knees back into your chest.

4 Repeat six times.

Focus points

- To make this exercise more challenging, lower your legs closer to the floor without touching it, and return your legs straight back to the vertical without bending, maintaining the contact of your back with the floor. If this contact cannot be maintained, you should continue to bend your knees until your strength has increased.

- If you cannot extend your legs to the vertical position, take your legs up a wall with your bottom as close to the wall as your flexibility will allow, making sure that your tailbone is on the floor. Keeping your tailbone on the floor, on an exhalation lift your legs away from the wall, keeping them straight. Hold the position as you inhale and then on the next exhalation release the legs on to the wall.

Half boat

Instructions

1 Sitting on the floor, bend your knees and hold the backs of your thighs.

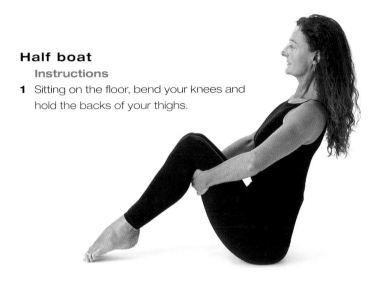

2 Keeping your back straight, your shoulders down and your chest lifted, lean back, resting the tips of your toes on the floor, and find your balance.

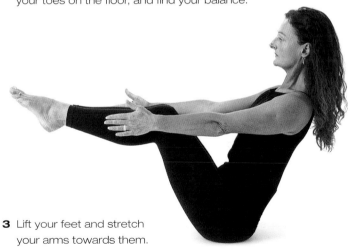

3 Lift your feet and stretch your arms towards them.

4 Hold for as long as you can and repeat three to six times.

Focus point

● Keep your back lifted and draw your abdomen in and up with each exhalation.

Cat pose

As well as lifting and toning the abdomen, this exercise also helps to keep the spine supple, relieving lower back pain and tension in the upper back and shoulders.

Instructions

1 Start on your hands and knees, with your back straight and the back of your head in line with your spine. Your hands should be underneath your shoulders and your knees below your hips.

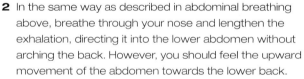

2 In the same way as described in abdominal breathing above, breathe through your nose and lengthen the exhalation, directing it into the lower abdomen without arching the back. However, you should feel the upward movement of the abdomen towards the lower back.

3 Inhale, maintaining the lift of the lower abdomen.

4 Repeat four to six times.

5 Continuing to breathe as above, on the next exhalation arch your back and at the same time move your chin to your chest, tucking in your tailbone.

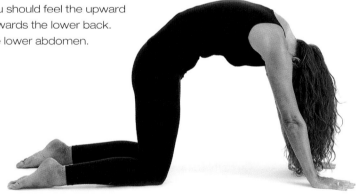

6 As you inhale lower the back a little, maintaining the lift on the abdomen.

7 On the next exhalation arch the back even farther.

8 Continue for another four to six breaths.

Focus points

- If you feel any pressure in your head take one or two normal breaths and then continue.
- Although you will feel the upper back stretching and opening, try to focus your attention on the lower back.

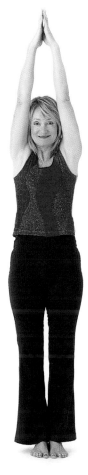

Half moon
This will also help keep your waist trim.

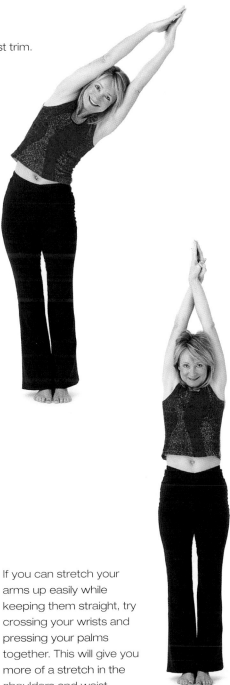

Instructions
1 Stand with your feet together, your legs straight and pulled up, and tailbone tucked in.

2 With an inhalation, stretch your arms up above your head and hook your thumbs.

3 Exhale and, keeping your tailbone in and your lower abdomen back, press your hips to the left as you stretch over to the right.

4 Stay in the position for one or two breaths, but without strain, then inhale and come up.
5 With an exhalation go to the left.
6 Repeat twice on both sides, staying longer and extending farther each time.

Focus points
- Be sure to keep the tailbone tucked in and the lower abdomen up and back throughout.
- As you extend to the right, keep your right hip forward in line with your left and take your left shoulder back in line with your right, and vice versa.
- If you can stretch your arms up easily while keeping them straight, try crossing your wrists and pressing your palms together. This will give you more of a stretch in the shoulders and waist.

Bridge

This is not an abdominal exercise, but complementary as it releases the abdomen and the back, and stretches the front hip area.

Instructions

1 Lie on your back with your knees bent and your feet flat on the floor hip-distance apart.

2 Place your hands palms down on the floor by your sides.

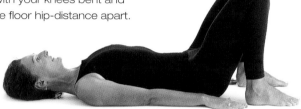

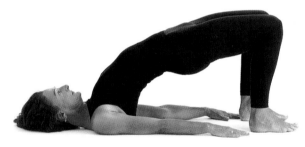

3 On an exhalation curl your pelvis away from the floor and continue to lift the front hips and the chest until all of your back is off the floor.

4 Roll your shoulders underneath you, so you are resting on the top most part of them. Interlace your fingers, stretching your shoulders, arms and knuckles towards your heels.

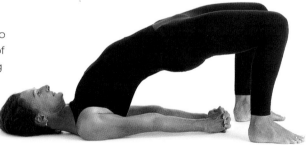

6 On an exhalation release your hands and shoulders and roll down slowly, placing the vertebrae on the floor one at a time.

7 Repeat once, changing the interlacing of your fingers.

Focus points

- Keeping your tailbone tucked in, move your breastbone towards your chin and stretch your thighs towards your knees.
- Do not let your knees move outwards and keep your feet parallel.

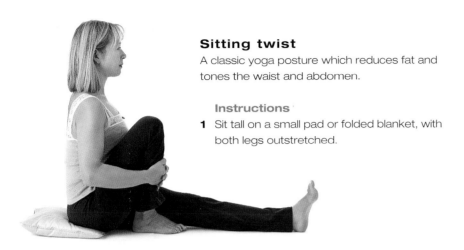

Sitting twist

A classic yoga posture which reduces fat and tones the waist and abdomen.

Instructions

1 Sit tall on a small pad or folded blanket, with both legs outstretched.

2 Keeping your left leg in place, bend your right leg, place the foot on the floor close to your right buttock and hold the top of your right shin with both hands. Lift your chest and extend your back upwards.

3 Turn to your right and hold the bent leg just below the knee with the crook of your left elbow. Place your right hand on the floor behind you, close to your left buttock.

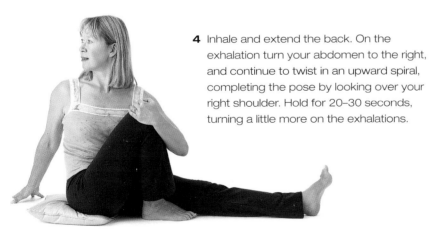

4 Inhale and extend the back. On the exhalation turn your abdomen to the right, and continue to twist in an upward spiral, completing the pose by looking over your right shoulder. Hold for 20–30 seconds, turning a little more on the exhalations.

5 Release and repeat on the other side.

Focus point

- Do not overturn the head, and keep the eyes and throat soft.
- Breathe softly and evenly throughout.

Lift and tone thighs and buttocks

Rather than clenching your buttocks, which only strengthens the 'clench', squat-based exercises increase the overall strength of buttocks and thighs, increasing lift and tone, and use the breath to hold rather than 'pulse'.

Squat sequence

Instructions

1 Stand with your feet parallel and hip-width apart.
2 Inhale, lifting your arms in front until they are horizontal.

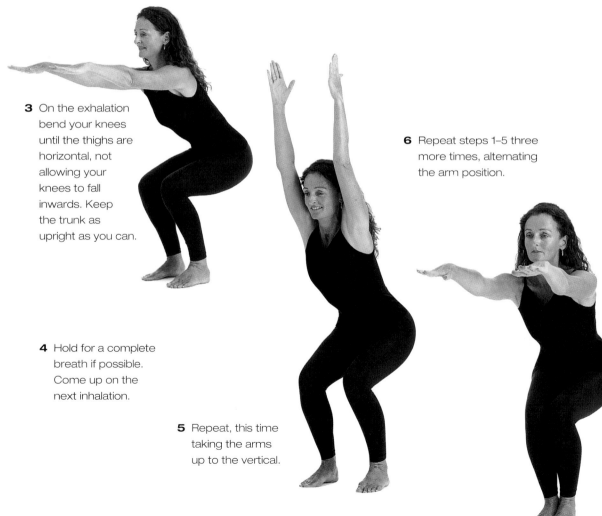

3 On the exhalation bend your knees until the thighs are horizontal, not allowing your knees to fall inwards. Keep the trunk as upright as you can.

6 Repeat steps 1–5 three more times, alternating the arm position.

4 Hold for a complete breath if possible. Come up on the next inhalation.

5 Repeat, this time taking the arms up to the vertical.

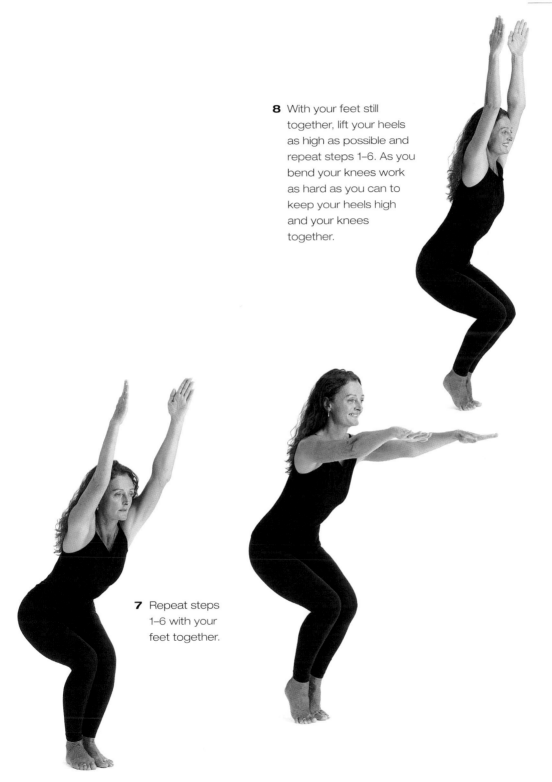

8 With your feet still together, lift your heels as high as possible and repeat steps 1–6. As you bend your knees work as hard as you can to keep your heels high and your knees together.

7 Repeat steps 1–6 with your feet together.

Warrior lunge

This exercise is essentially a combination of two yoga poses – the warrior and the triangle.

Instructions

1 Stand with your feet parallel and 3–4 feet apart, hands on hips.
2 Turn your right leg and foot 90 degrees out, so that the knee and big toe point directly to your right. Keep your hips and chest facing forward and take your tailbone in.

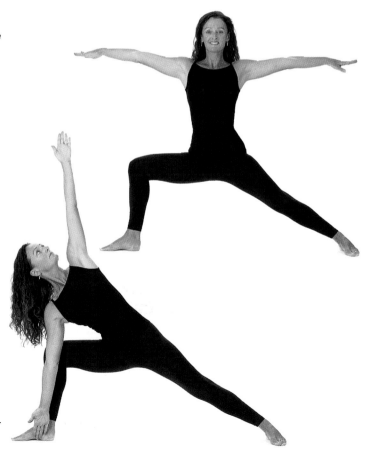

3 Inhale, lift your chest, and on the exhalation bend your right leg towards your little toe until the shin is vertical.

4 Hold for a breath or two. On an inhalation straighten the leg, turn the feet back to parallel and repeat to the left.
5 Repeat 1–3. Continue to bend the leg farther to bring the thigh closer to the horizontal.
6 Stretch your arms out sideways. Inhale, stretch to your right and bring your right elbow to the inside of your right knee, stretching your hand towards your right ankle, and stretching your left arm upwards. Do not rest your elbow on your knee, and do not place your hand on the floor. Look up to the top hand and hold for a breath or two.
7 Repeat to the left.

Focus points

- The width of your starting stride depends on the length of your legs. To test the distance go into the pose. Your shin should be vertical and, eventually, your thigh horizontal.
- Keep the breath even and soft.

Bridge leg lift

This exercise has a toning and lifting effect on thighs and buttocks similar to that of squat-based exercises, but works by strengthening and elongating the front thighs.

Instructions

1 Lie on your back with your knees bent, feet together and shins vertical. Place your arms by your sides, palms facing down.

2 Tilt your pelvis and lift your back, keeping your tailbone in, and draw your abdomen towards your back.

3 Press your left foot into the floor, keeping your left knee in over the ankle. Bend your right knee into your chest and extend the leg vertically to the ceiling. Hold for two to three breaths.

4 Repeat on the other side.

5 If you find the exercise easy and you want to increase the intensity, lower the lifted leg on an exhalation until it is parallel with the thigh of the bent leg. On an inhalation return to vertical. Repeat three to four times on each side.

Focus points

- Do not hold your breath – your breathing should be soft and even.
- Keep your hips level.

Hip openers and leg releases

Keeping the hip, knee and ankle joints supple will also help to improve circulation and lymphatic flow, and improve appearance and posture. The sitting or kneeling positions provide ideal opportunities to implement other anti-ageing strategies such as facial exercises and meditation. Alternatively relax with a book or watch television. The longer you stay in these positions, the more beneficial they are.

Crossed-legged sitting forward

This position stretches the buttocks and releases the hips and lower back.

Instructions

1 Sit on the floor in the simple cross-legged position or the half lotus position (*see* pages 45 and 123).

2 On an inhalation lift your chest and extend your back. Exhale and bring your hands forward beyond your shins. Inhale once again to extend the back farther up, and with the exhalation go forward, stretching the arms as far away from the hips as you can.

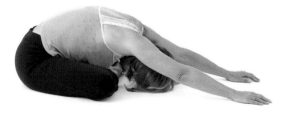

3 To rest in the position, bend the elbows and place your chin in your hands.
4 Stay as long as you can, then change the cross of your legs and repeat.

Focus points

- Concentrate on going forward to extend the back rather than trying to get your head on the floor.
- Keep your breathing soft and even, and try to 'let go' during the exhalation.

Supine crossed legs

This opens the front of the hips and releases the groin.

Instructions

1 Sit on the floor in the simple cross-legged position (*see* page 45).

2 Lean back onto your elbows, and lift your buttocks slightly to lengthen your lower back. Roll your back down, removing your elbows and resting your head on the floor.

3 Rest in the position for up to two minutes, then change the cross of your legs and repeat.

4 You can combine this hip opener with a shoulder release by holding the elbows and taking the arms over the head.

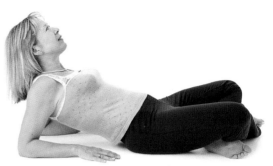

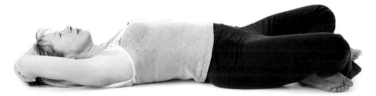

Focus point

• Keep your tailbone in to ensure your back remains long.

The cobbler

Another classic yoga position which has many benefits for the organs of the lower abdomen and is excellent for the knees, hips and pelvic joints.

Instructions

1 Sit on the floor and bring the soles of your feet together. If you cannot straighten your back, sit up against a wall or use a small pad or folded blanket for support.

2 Hold your toes or your ankles and lift your chest. Extend your knees away from your hips and towards the floor.

3 Stay in the position for up to five minutes.

Focus points

• Keep the feet close to the pubic bone.
• Try to relax the groin.

Supine cobbler

This position has the same benefits as the cobbler.

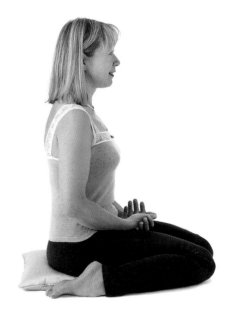

Instructions

1 Sit on the floor with the soles of your feet together, as above, but without support.
2 Lean back onto your elbows. Lift your buttocks slightly and move them closer to your heels, and lengthen your lower back. Roll your back down, removing your elbows and resting your head on the floor.
3 Rest the arms on the floor, palms up.

Kneeling hero

This is very good for the circulation and for lymphatic flow in the legs.

Instructions

1 Kneel up on the floor with your knees together and your feet a little wider than your hips.
2 Use the tips of your fingers to take the calf muscles down towards the heels, and roll them very slightly out.
3 Sit down in between your heels and remove your fingers. If your buttocks do not reach the floor you will need a support such as a folded blanket, pad or telephone directory.
4 Stay for five minutes or as long as you feel able, then stretch your legs forward, pressing your knees to the floor.

Focus points

- This position stretches the knees, but you should not feel pain in them. If you do, come out of the position or try sitting higher.
- If your ankles are stiff, place a rolled blanket or towel underneath the ankle joint.

Bowing kneeling hero

This increases mobility of the hips and releases
the lower back.

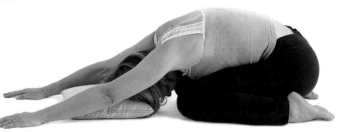

Instructions

1 Kneel as above, placing your hands
   on the floor in front of the knees.
2 Sliding your hands forward, slowly
   take your head down.
3 Hold as long as you feel able.

Focus points

- Try to keep your buttocks down.
- If you cannot rest your head on the floor, rest it on a support.
- Allow your knees to separate a little.

Victory pose

So-called because of the V shape of the legs, and reflecting the
achievement of mastering it!

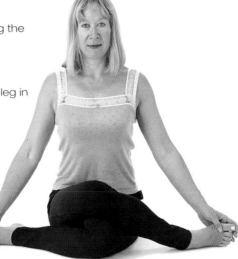

Instructions

1 Sit on the floor in a cross-legged position with your right leg in
   front.
2 Slide your left foot farther around towards your right
   buttock, then bring your right foot around to your left
   buttock. Your legs should form a symmetrical V shape
   with your knees at its apex.
3 Inhale, lift your chest, and on the exhalation take
   your hands forward in front of the knees and
   slide as far forward as you can.
4 Hold as long as you are able, then reverse legs.

Focus points

- If you cannot get into the position, try sitting on a support.
- Aim to take the top knee directly over the bottom knee.
- Keep both buttocks on the floor.

Variations

All of the sitting and kneeling positions can be combined with a twist
as described in the Sitting twist (see page 89), or forward bend.

97

Tone and shape flabby arms

As you age the skin and muscle of the upper arm seems to dissociate itself from the bone, and the prospect of wearing strappy tops can be daunting. The following exercises will lift, tone and shape your arms and chest, and strengthen elbows and wrists.

Press ups

The classic way to strengthen and tone your arms and lift your bust.

Instructions (easier version)

1 Begin on all fours, with your hands slightly in front of your shoulders and pointing straight forwards, and your knees beneath your hips.
2 On an exhalation bend your elbows back towards your knees as if to take your forearms to the floor. Keep the elbows in and the hands flat. On the inhalation push up slowly.
3 Now turn your hands inwards. Repeat as above, this time bending your elbows out.
4 Repeat the sequence three to four times.

Focus points

- Breathe slowly and softly.
- Keep your tailbone in and your shoulders away from your ears.
- To increase the intensity, move the hands farther forwards.

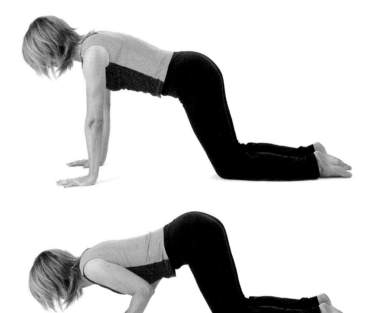

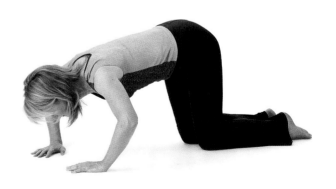

Instructions (harder version)

1 Begin on all fours again, but with your hands farther forward, so that when you tuck your toes under, lift your knees and straighten your legs, your arms will be vertical.
2 On an exhalation bend your elbows. On the inhalation push up slowly.
3 Repeat three to four times or as many times as you can.

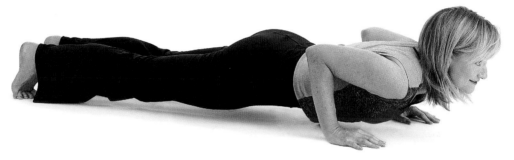

Focus points

• Keep your legs straight and your heels stretching back.
• Keep your tailbone in and lift your abdomen towards your back.
• Keep the breathing soft and even. If it becomes strained, stop and rest. Try again when your breathing is quiet – as your stamina builds up you will be able to do more.

Tricep dips

Targets the underarm area.

Instructions

1 Sit forward on a stable chair with your hands holding the front edge.
2 Slide your bottom off the edge of the chair so that your legs make a 90 degree angle at the knees.
3 On an exhalation bend your elbows back, lowering your bottom towards the floor until your arms make a 90 degree angle at the elbows.)
4 On the inhalation straighten your arms.
5 Repeat three or four times, or as many as you can.

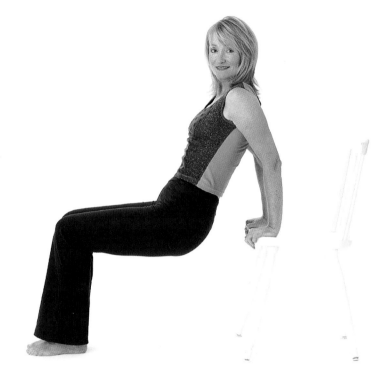

Focus point

• Keep your shoulders away from your ears.

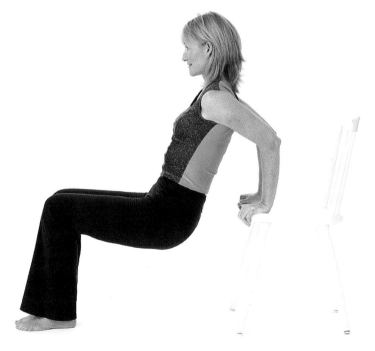

The crow

This yoga posture, which takes its name from the feet of the crow, strengthens the arms, wrists, shoulders and abdomen.

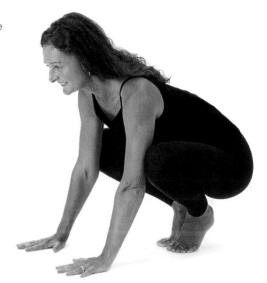

Instructions

1 Squat with the knees wide and place your hands shoulder-width apart on the floor in between your knees. Spread your fingers out like the feet of a crow.
2 Lift your heels and bend your elbows as you place your inner knees on the outer upper arms.
3 Lift your head and focus your eyes on a point ahead.

4 Move your weight forward onto your hands. Find your balance and lift your feet.
5 Pressing your hands into the floor, lift your hips and your head, and slowly straighten your arms as much as you can. Hold for as long as you can, breathing softly and deeply.

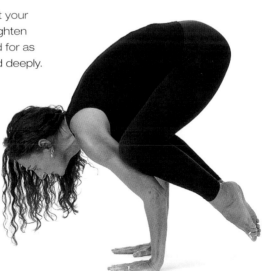

Focus points

- If you cannot lift both feet, try lifting one at a time.
- Do not drop the head.
- Grip the upper arms with the knees.

Arm and shoulder release

Stiff, hunched shoulders also add years to your appearance. The following exercises will relieve stiffness and tension. These exercises are especially beneficial for RSI (Repetitive Strain Injury) sufferers.

Breathe into your shoulders

Moving with your breath helps release tension and stiffness.

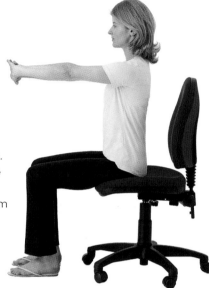

Instructions

1 Sit with your back straight, your chest lifted and your shoulders rolling back. Move your abdomen back and up. Have your feet hip-distance apart with your toes pointing straight forward. If your feet are not firmly flat on the ground place books beneath them.

2 Interlace your fingers. Exhale and press the hands forwards horizontally away from your chest, turning your palms out and then straightening your arms.

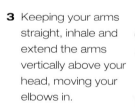

3 Keeping your arms straight, inhale and extend the arms vertically above your head, moving your elbows in.

4 Exhale, keep your hands above your head and bend the elbows out to the sides. Resting your hands on the crown of your head, take your shoulders down and extend the elbows away from one other.

5 Inhale and extend the arms above your head. Press the thumb side of your hand up higher than the little-finger side.

6 Exhale and take your arms forward.

7 Repeat several times in a continuous movement, changing the interlacing of your fingers halfway through so that the other hand is on top.

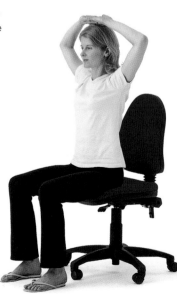

Focus points

- Keep your chest lifted, even when bringing your arms down.
- Breathe through your nose without holding your breath. Your breathing should be soft, slow, deep and rhythmic.

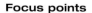

Chest opener

This exercise opens your chest, relieves stiffness in your shoulders and upper back, and improves posture.

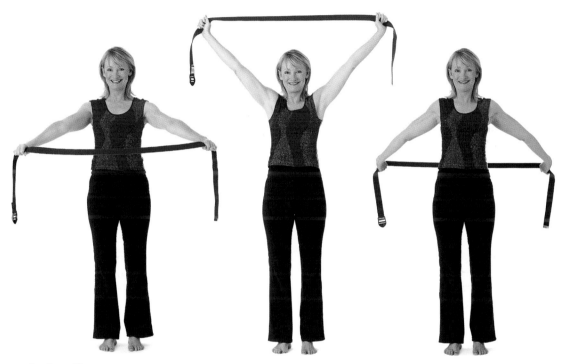

Instructions

1 Hold a belt or length of cord in both hands, approximately two shoulder-widths apart.

2 Keeping your arms straight, breathe in and take your arms up above your head, keeping the belt stretched.

3 Breathe out and take the belt over your head and round to the back.

4 Breathe in and lift the belt back up.

5 Breathing out, lower the arms over to the front so that you have made a full circle.

6 Repeat up to five times.

Focus points

- Make the movement soft, slow and fluid.
- Keep your chest lifted, your shoulders down and your tailbone in.
- If you do not feel the stretch, bring your hands closer together.

103

Three-point arm stretch

This exercise stretches the whole of the arm, improves flexibility in the wrists and shoulders, and also includes a back stretch. It is, however, harder than it looks.

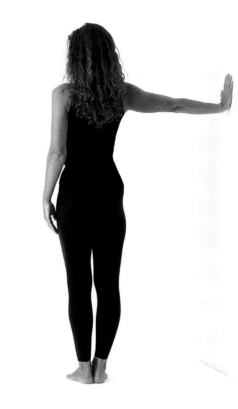

Instructions

1 Stand with your right side next to a wall, about one and a half to two feet away, and place your right hand flat on the wall at shoulder level, with your fingers stretching upwards.

2 Keeping contact with the wall, step away until the arm is straight. Stand upright, without leaning into the hand, and keep your shoulders down. Hold for two or three breaths.

3 Keeping the right hand in place, turn towards the wall and place the left hand parallel to the right hand, shoulder-width apart.

4 Press your hands into the wall and walk your feet back until your legs are vertical. Stretch your hips and thighs back away from the wall and your heels into the floor.

5 Hold for two to three breaths.

6 Walk in, then, keeping your left hand to the wall, repeat on the left side.

7 Repeat the whole sequence two to three times.

Focus point

• When you have one hand to the wall, try to roll the shoulders back and down. If this is hard, turn the hand 90 degrees so the fingers point backwards. This is another valuable way of working in the sequence.

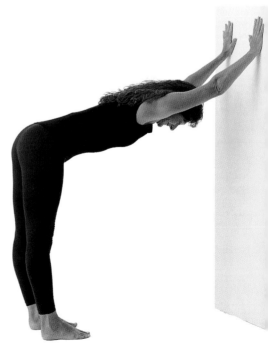

The Anchor

This position improves circulation and flexibility
in the upper back, shoulders and neck.

Instructions

1 Kneel with your legs together, your buttocks
on your heels and your head on the floor

2 Interlace your fingers behind your back.

3 On an inhalation, stretch your knuckles
away from your shoulders. As you
exhale lift your hands, arms and
shoulders upwards, eventually
up as far as the vertical
and beyond.

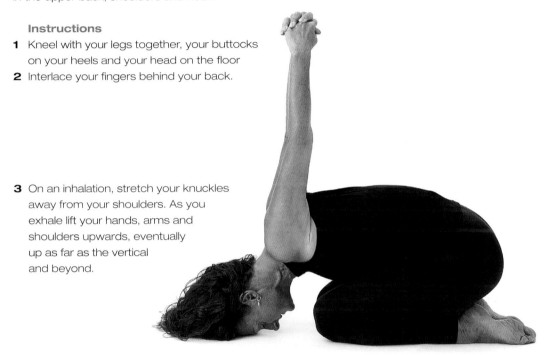

4 Hold for two to three breaths or as long as you can.
Repeat, changing the interlacing of your fingers.

Gravity-defying exercises: suggested sequences

The following six sequences take approximately ten minutes each, depending on the number of repetitions done. The first three sequences are mixed, and will help lift and tone your abdomen, thighs, buttocks and arms, whilst the next three target specific parfts of the body. For a good balance use a different sequence each day of the week, with one day a week off.

Sequence 1 (mixed)

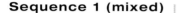

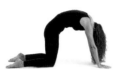

Cat pose with abdominal breathing (page 86)

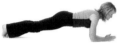

Elbow lift (page 83)

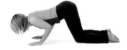

Press ups (easy version) (page 98)

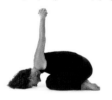

Anchor (page 105)

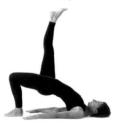

Bridge leg lift (page 93)

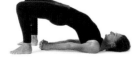

Bridge (page 88)

Sequence 2 (mixed)

Squat sequence (page 90)

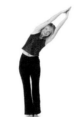

Half moon (page 87)

Crow (page 101)

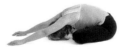

Cross-legged sitting forward (page 94)

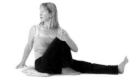

Sitting twist (page 89)

Supine crossed legs (page 95)

Sequence 3 (mixed)

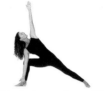

Warrior lunge (page 92)

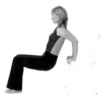

Tricep dips (page 100)

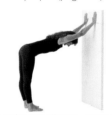

Three-point arm stretch (page 104)

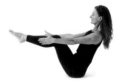

Half Boat (page 85)

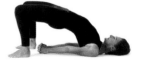

Bridge (page 88)

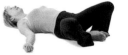

Supine cobbler (page 96)

Sequence 4 (abdominals)

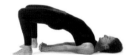

Abdominal breathing   (page 82)

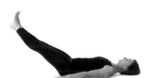

Pelvic tilts   (page 83)

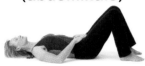

Leg lowering   (page 84)

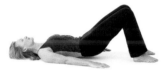

Bridge   (page 88)

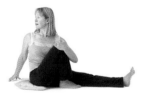

Sitting twist   (page 89)

Supine crossed legs   (page 95)

Sequence 5 (thighs and buttocks)

Squat sequence   (page 90)

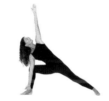

Warrior lunge   (page 92)

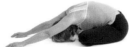

Bowing kneeling hero (arms stretched forward) (page 97)

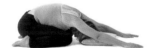

Cross-legged sitting forward (page 94)

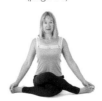

Victory pose   (page 97)

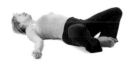

Supine cobbler   (page 96)

Sequence 6 (arms)

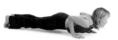

Press ups   (page 99)

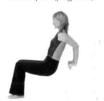

Tricep dips   (page 100)

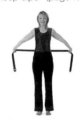

Chest opener   (page 103)

Breathe into your shoulders   (page 102)

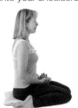

As above in kneeling hero   (page 96)

Anchor   (page 105)

hand care

Next to the face, the hands are arguably the most expressive part of the body, and elegant, well-manicured hands a tremendous physical asset. Hands and nails speak volumes about a person's health and the importance they place on personal grooming, and are often said to be the truest indication of age.

But though circulatory problems can cause puffy hands and poor skin tone, and arthritis results in stiffness of the joints, much ageing of the hands is premature and avoidable, the result of inadequate care and protection, and being constantly in the line of fire. Exposing your hands to all kinds of weather conditions from severe cold to strong sunlight without barrier creams or sunscreen eventually results in liver spots, slackening of the skin and wrinkles. Similarly, using your hands without the protection of gloves for household and other chores causes rough, dry skin and brittle, flaking nails. Because they are in frequent use, hands are also susceptible to injury – cuts, burns and so on – which take more time to heal if your skin is dry and damaged.

The good news is that even neglected hands respond surprisingly well to a little tender loving care. Not everyone has the good fortune to be born with perfectly shaped hands, but most people can achieve healthy, attractive-looking hands without too much effort by following a few basic rules and giving themselves a weekly ten-minute manicure.

Routine hand care

- Always wear appropriate gloves when out and about in cold weather, gardening, and for household tasks, especially those that involve immersing your hands in water, or contact with detergents and other cleansing agents.
- Use a good handcream to moisturize your hands and always reapply after washing and last thing at night. Have it to hand at every sink and basin in the house, at work, in the car, in your handbag. A retinol-based handcream may help to reduce signs of ageing, but be sure it contains a sunscreen, or that you use a sunscreen with it during daylight hours.
- Use only mild soap, if any.
- Always dry hands well, especially between the fingers.
- Wear nail varnish by all means, but not all the time. Like skin, nails need to breathe.

Ten-minute manicure

1 Remove any nail varnish.

2 Soak your hands for a couple of minutes in a bowl of warm (not hot) water to which you have added a good pinch of sea salt, a few drops of essential oils such as lavender or peppermint or, if they need a good scrub, any commercially available cleanser that will not dry them out.

3 Dry hands well and gently push back unruly cuticles with a flannel, towel or your fingertips.

4 Trim your nails straight across, preferably using nail pliers (available in any good chemist) rather than clippers or scissors. Finish and shape using an emery board, always filing from the side to the centre of the nail.

5 Moisturize with handcream, giving your hands a massage as you do so. Using a circular motion, rub cream into your fingers using the thumb of the opposite hand, working from the fingertips to the knuckles, and then with a firm movement of the thumbs move down the back of the hand to the wrist.

6 Allow your fingernails to be free of nail varnish at least half the time, but if you wish to apply varnish at the end of your manicure, first remove any residue of oil with a pad of cotton wool moistened with nail varnish remover. Apply a base coat before painting with varnish.

feet

Our feet are an incredible piece of precision engineering, each foot made up of no fewer than 26 bones – that's an eighth of the total number in the whole skeleton – and designed for bearing both the weight of the body and propelling it forward. Over a lifetime our feet will carry us an estimated 70,000 miles, around 18,000 steps each day. Yet our feet are one of the most neglected and abused parts of the body. We take them for granted and subject them to incredible pressures, teetering around in ill-fitting shoes and killer heels.

Walking barefoot is your best insurance against the development of foot problems, which are rare in societies where shoes are not worn, but unpractical in the Western world. Sensible shoes are the next best alternative but any styles which give the feet some support and have heels less than two inches high are better than slip-ons and high heels. If you are a shoe-aholic with a penchant for strappy sandals and pointy toes with four-inch stiletto heels, reserve them for special occasions. Glamorous they may be, but the price of sexy spikes is prematurely aged and damaged feet, and a whole host of other health problems – twisted ankles, damaged knee joints, back pain, neck pain, headaches and poor posture for starters. Add to that the pained expression and physical tension that hobbling around in uncomfortable, ill-fitting shoes cause, and it is easy to see how they can add years to your appearance.

Feet age in various ways, partly due to genetic inheritance and partly to the way we treat them, and most often a combination of both. Looking after your feet not only keeps them looking and feeling good, it makes a major difference to your quality of life in later years. Damaged feet are literally disabling, causing anything from discomfort when you walk to severely restricting your ability to do so.

Structural damage to the feet as a result of ageing can be caused by osteoporosis, which increases the risk of fractures, and bunions, a preventable form of arthritis causing unsightly and painful lumps at the joint at the base of the big toe. Narrow shoes with pointed toes and high heels throw the weight forwards onto the balls of the feet and overload the 'bunion' joints, making them rub against the shoe causing bunions to form, and speeding up their development in people with a genetic predisposition. Small bunions can be treated by wearing well-fitting shoes and corrective insoles or toe pads. Larger bunions require surgery.

Ageing also affects the skin covering the foot. Skin on the soles of the feet is much thicker and tougher than that covering the rest of the body, but with age it often becomes harder and drier, resulting in unattractively cracked heels, especially in summer when the feet are more exposed. Ill-fitting shoes result in corns and calluses – thick layers of skin formed by the feet to protect them against pressure and rubbing.

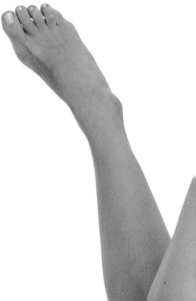

Like hands, feet respond well to a little care and attention. Even if you never achieve model feet you can certainly achieve well-cared-for feet that look and feel good. If you have any foot problems visit a chiropodist to sort them out and maintain the health of your feet by following the advice below and combining it with a ten-minute pedicure once or twice a week.

Routine foot care

- Invest in a variety of comfortable, supportive and well-fitting shoes to suit different purposes – trainers for exercising, walking shoes for a hike across the moors – and yes, strappy sandals with spikey heels for hot dates.
- Take regular brisk walks to exercise the feet in the way they were designed for, keep your circulation going and reduce your risk of osteoporosis. If walking hurts your feet, get advice from a chiropodist.
- Maintain good posture (*see* the body check on page 67). Wearing well-fitting shoes will help to distribute weight evenly over the feet.
- Increase flexibility by rotating the ankles in each direction, and up and down, and by rolling the feet to and fro over an empty wine bottle or similar.
- Lavish as much care on your feet as you do on your face, soaking them regularly and moisturizing daily, avoiding the area between the toes.
- Always dry feet carefully, especially between the toes.
- To soften the skin, apply Vaseline or deep moisturizing cream then put on a pair of socks to sleep in.

Ten-minute pedicure

1 Remove any nail varnish.
2 Soak your feet for a couple of minutes in a bowl of warm (not hot) water to which you have added a good pinch of sea salt, a few drops of essential oils such as lavender or peppermint or, if they need a good scrub, any commercially available cleanser that will not dry them out.
3 Dry feet well and gently push back unruly cuticles with a flannel, towel or your fingertips.
4 Trim your nails straight across, preferably using nail pliers (available in any good chemist) rather than clippers or scissors. Nails on the feet tend to become thicker with age and when very thick can create a lot of pressure, so if yours are thickening, gently file the top surface or have it done professionally.
5 Buff the skin using a foot file or rough skin remover.
6 Apply a deep moisturizing cream – feet have more layers of dead skin than the rest of the body so need a richer moisturizer – giving your feet a massage with your thumbs as you do so.
7 If you wish, apply varnish at the end of your pedicure in the same way as for a manicure (*see* page 109)

mind & spirit

Optimism and enthusiasm are super-young characteristics, and everyone likes being around people who are upbeat and cheerful. Their positive energy rubs off on us and recharges our batteries. Unsurprisingly, optimists are known to live longer on average than pessimists, and they almost invariably look younger than their peers. By contrast negativity, in all its forms, is ageing. No one wants to spend time with miseries who drone on about their problems and what's wrong with the world. It's too draining. But can pessimists change the way they think?

Research shows they can, though it takes effort and commitment. Page 41 outlines the principles of positive thinking and changing negative thought patterns, but devoting ten minutes to almost any of the techniques described throughout Part 3 will help you acquire a more positive outlook. Meditation is particularly beneficial. Be open-minded, if you cannot be optimistic, about the likelihood of success and your chances increase. The good news is that the more positive you are, the more positive you become. It's an upward and empowering cycle.

One of the things that most concerns people as they grow older is loss of memory and brain power. Like physical performance, mental abilities tend to deteriorate with age, but not as much or as frequently as many people fear. Lifestyle choices have been found to protect against and even reverse mild age-related memory loss and mental decline. Genetic predisposition affects your risk of developing more severe forms of memory loss such as Alzheimer's, but even so lifestyle plays an equal part in determining your risk. Prevention, rather than cure, is the key. Strategies that protect your brain include: a healthy diet high in antioxidants (*see* pages 20–21); supplementation with the antioxidant vitamins E and C, and folic acid; hormone therapy; regular physical exercise including aerobic activity (and excluding sports and activities that increase your risk of serious head injuries); yoga, in particular inverted postures such as the headstand and shoulderstand; keeping yourself stimulated mentally and intellectually; being involved in constructive, meaningful activities; relieving and controlling stress.

As well as being detrimental to brain health and associated with memory loss, chronic stress is ageing in other ways. First of all it makes you look older, contributing to the formation of frown and worry lines, and to facial tension, and often leads to poor posture which can add another ten years onto your appearance. More insidious still is its effect on your health. Unrelieved stress doubles your chances of coronary heart disease and causes hypertension, migraines and insomnia. Chronically stressed individuals who use cigarettes and too much alcohol to relax only exacerbate the problem in the long run, as well as adding to their wrinkle quota.

The strategies in the following pages include relaxation techniques for effective stress relief and a variety of meditation techniques. Regular meditation has been dubbed the 'relaxation response' and is known to have remarkable anti-ageing benefits, both physically and mentally (*see* pages 44–45). As welll as keeping stress at bay and bringing peace of mind, it sharpens the intellect, promotes emotional clarity, increases optimism and brings enormous spiritual benefits.

mental exercise

People who are intellectually active throughout their lives – who achieve higher educational attainments, spend time reading, keep on learning, have stimulating jobs and so on – have a much lower risk of mental deterioration and memory loss as they age. Mental activity – exercising your brain in a variety of ways – increases the density of neural connections in the brain, improving memory and reducing your risk of future mental decline.

Test your memory using the word list below. Set a timer for one minute while you study the words. When the minute is up, set the timer for 20 minutes while you go about your normal business. When the 20 minutes are up, write down as many of the words as you can. Remembering fewer than half the words on the list is an indication that you need to work on boosting your memory. If you are less than happy with your result, take action now. Keep your brain in shape by cultivating various interests and hobbies, enrolling on courses and learning new skills. Stretch your mind with regular ten-minute mental workouts such as the following:

- take up a musical instrument and practise for ten minutes daily
- spend ten minutes a day learning a language – book up a holiday to encourage you
- do crosswords and other puzzles
- play chess and other games of skill
- memorize lists of words – English or in a foreign language – telephone numbers, poems and so on
- at checkout counters do a little mental arithmetic, working out the total costs of your groceries in your head

WORD LIST

peach	knee
pollution	grass
insect	radiator
cottage	chairman
shawl	oil

deep relaxation

Chronic stress is the enemy of youth, but you can break through the stress cycle by taking the right action. By doing so you will take a major step towards improving the health of both your body and your brain, and smooth out the ageing worry lines that high levels of unrelieved stress cause.

Yoga and meditation are excellent ways to turn off the flow of stress hormones – adrenalin, noradrenalin and cortisol – which circulate through the bloodstream when we are stressed. The relaxation and deep breathing they promote switch on the parasympathetic nervous system, which reverses the stress response and activates the body's healing mechanisms.

The following technique, which is based on yoga, completely relaxes the mind and body by progressively releasing muscular tension in each and every part of the body. As you let go of physical tension, the mind automatically relaxes and becomes quiet. Relaxing in this way destroys fatigue and alleviates stress and stress-related symptoms such as headaches, migraine, insomnia and memory impairment.

You may find it helpful to record the instructions below, leaving a sufficient pause in which to relax each body part before moving on to the next.

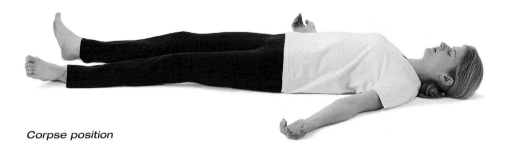

Corpse position

Instructions

1 Lie flat on your back in the corpse position (*see* page 115).

2 Close your eyes and focus on your breathing. Take a few slow, deep abdominal breaths (*see* opposite). Inhale to a count of four, exhale to a count of four, then allow your breathing to settle into a light, even, relaxed rhythm.

3 Now turn your attention to releasing tension by consciously relaxing each part of the body in turn. First bring your attention to your feet for a few moments and send them the message to let go. Relax them as deeply as you can and then move your awareness to your calves and repeat the process.

4 Work your way up the body in the same fashion, relaxing your thighs, buttocks, hips, abdomen, lower back, chest, upper back, hands, forearms, upper arms, shoulders, throat, neck and head.

5 Pay special attention to the subtle art of relaxing your face. Relax your jaw and mouth, allowing your lips to part slightly and your tongue to rest in the lower half of your mouth. Soften and relax your cheeks. Relax your eyes, allowing them to sink back into their sockets. Relax your brows, forehead and temples. Feel your skin softening over your features as your facial muscles completely relax. Finally relax your scalp and all the muscles in your head.

6 Scan your entire body from the tips of your toes to the top of your scalp. Breathe into any remaining pockets of tension. Let go and relax as you breathe out.

7 You are now completely relaxed. As the full weight of your body rests on the floor feel yourself sinking into the ground.

8 Breathing normally, maintain awareness of your breathing, gently bringing your attention back to it when your mind wanders. Remain in this position for five or ten minutes.

9 To come out of the position gently bring your knees to your chest and roll over onto one side. Rest on your side for a few moments and then, when you are ready, get up.

breath control

Breath is our life force. As long as there is breath in the body, there is life, and regulating the breathing process is an effective way to boost mental and physical health and relaxation. It is also considered a powerful tool in spiritual development, so much so that an entire branch of yoga is devoted to the art and science of breath control, through which it is said one may attain immortality, and many forms of meditation involve breath awareness.

Animals and children instinctively breathe correctly, but without our being aware of it we tend to breathe less efficiently as we become adult, using only the upper part of the chest. Generally when we are calm and relaxed we breathe deeply, in a slow and rhythmic fashion. When anxious and stressed we breathe faster, with shallow, irregular breaths sometimes punctuated by gasps as our bodies strive to increase the supply of oxygen. If this pattern of breathing continues unchecked it becomes a habit, which in turn makes us more nervous and agitated, and a vicious circle is established.

Simply by becoming aware of your breathing you can begin to reverse bad habits and train yourself to breathe correctly. The technique of abdominal breathing described below also helps correct shallow breathing and is an effective way to relax.

Abdominal breathing

Abdominal breathing is a way of breathing using the abdominal muscles, as the name suggests, and encouraging movement of the diaphragm, allowing the lungs to fill to capacity and expel air more efficiently.

Instructions

1 Stretch out on your back in the corpse position (*see* page 115).
2 Close your eyes and breathe in slowly and evenly through your nostrils. Feel your abdomen swelling and rising, then your ribcage expanding and finally your upper chest filling with air. Pause briefly before breathing out fully.
3 As you release the breath note the reverse movement. Feel your abdomen falling, the ribcage contracting, and finally the upper chest lowering as the air is expelled. Pause briefly before breathing in again.
4 Repeat this cycle in a flowing, steady movement for a few minutes and then let your breathing return to normal.

To establish the habit of breathing deeply and healthily, focus your attention several times a day on your breathing – you can be lying down, sitting up, standing or walking around – and consciously breathe from the abdomen for a minute or two.

Complete breathing

In complete breathing you make full use of your lungs, though never to the point of strain or discomfort. This is a yogic technique similar to abdominal breathing, but instead of lying on your back you sit upright, which allows more air to be drawn in and produces a fuller sensation.

Complete breathing calms and steadies the mind, and energizes the whole system. It also relieves anxiety, lifts depression, and promotes clear and positive thinking. Once the technique has been mastered, it can be used at will in any circumstances for instant stress relief.

Instructions

1 Sit in any crossed-legged position keeping your back comfortably straight. Breathe in and out through your nostrils throughout.
2 Now visualize your lungs as having three spaces – lower, middle and upper – and inhalation as happening in the three stages (steps 3–5) that follow.
3 As you begin to draw in air, the diaphragm pushes downwards into the abdomen, causing it to swell out as the lower space is filled.
4 As you continue to inhale, the ribcage expands as air is drawn into the middle space.
5 As you complete the inhalation, the upper chest broadens (but note that the shoulders are not lifted) as the upper space is filled with air.
6 When your lungs feel comfortably full, hold the breath for a few seconds, then exhale in a smooth, continuous movement.
7 As you exhale, the air leaves the lower lungs first, then the middle, and then the upper lungs.
8 Make four or five complete in-and-out breaths (taking about a minute), then breathe normally (abdominally) for half a minute, then do four or five more complete breaths.

Focus points

- Although the inhalation is visualized as happening in three stages, it should be a smooth, continuous movement.
- As you inhale, visualize yourself breathing in energy. As you exhale, visualize yourself breathing out tension and fatigue.
- Once you have grasped the movement, practise in an even, rhythmic fashion. To begin with keep to a ratio between inhalation, retention and exhalation of 1:1:1, to a count of about four for each inhalation. Then move on to a ration of 1:1:2, so if you inhale and hold to a count of four, you then exhale to a count of eight. Follow with alternate nostril breathing and/or meditation.

Alternate nostril breathing

Alternate nostril breathing is another yogic method of breath control which has a very calming, relaxing effect and is especially helpful for people who suffer from insomnia.

Instructions

1 Sit in any crossed-legged position keeping your back comfortably straight.
2 Fold the index and middle fingers of your right hand into your palm and lift it up to your nose. Close your eyes.

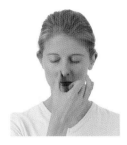 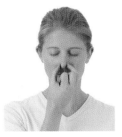 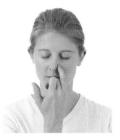

3 Close your right nostril with your thumb and exhale through the left, and then inhale fully to a count of four.

4 Keeping your right nostril blocked, close the left with your ring and little fingers, and hold your breath to a count of 16.

5 Release your thumb and breathe out through your right nostril to a count of eight. Still keeping your left nostril closed, inhale fully to a count of four.

6 Keeping your left nostril blocked, close the right nostril with your thumb, and hold your breath to a count of 16.
7 Release your ring and little fingers and breathe out through your left nostril to a count of eight. This completes one round. Start with two or three rounds and build up to 10.

Focus points

- The traditional ratio between inhalation, retention and exhalation is 1:4:2, but to avoid strain beginners are advised to keep to a ratio of 1:2:2, 1:1:2 or 1:1:1.
- Breathe smoothly and slowly, using the abdomen, throughout, and keep your facial muscles relaxed.
- As you breathe, focus your attention on the space in between your eyebrows. Follow with a few minutes' meditation.

Bellows breathing

Bellows breathing, or bhastrika, is a powerful yogic breathing technique used to still the mind in preparation for meditation. It is also said to purify the body, improving digestion and helping with the elimination of waste products, and strengthen the abdominal muscles. Above all it is highly regarded by yogis as a potent way to arouse latent spiritual forces.

In this technique the breath is controlled entirely by rapid movements of the abdominal muscles, so it is best to master the technique of abdominal breathing (*see* page 82) before attempting it. If you practise bellows breathing incorrectly, using your stomach instead of your abdominal muscles, you are liable to experience dizziness or nausea. Because bellows breathing is an intense and very vigorous technique, it is not suitable for people with heart, lung, eye or ear problems, with high or low blood pressure, or for pregnant women.

Bellows breathing should be practised on an empty stomach in an airy environment. Wait at least two hours after a light meal, five or six after a heavy one, before doing it and then another half-hour afterwards before eating again.

Instructions

1 Sit in any crossed-legged position keeping your back comfortably straight.
2 Begin breathing in and out rapidly through the nose by contracting the abdominal muscles quickly and forcibly, then immediately relaxing them again so that air is automatically drawn back into the lungs.
3 Continue rhythmically for ten breaths, gradually increasing to about 20 as you get more used to the exercise.
4 On the final exhalation contract the abdomen fully and empty the lungs completely.
5 Take in a slow, deep abdominal breath, and hold it as long as you comfortably can.
6 Exhale completely.
7 This completes one round of bellows breathing. Repeat two or three times, resting in between each round with a few normal breaths.

Lie in the corpse pose (*see* page 115) for a few minutes until your breathing has become quiet and still, or sit for meditation.

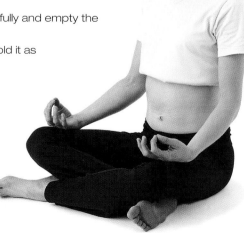

meditation techniques

The remarkable anti-ageing benefits of regular meditation have been described in Part 2 (*see* pages 44–45). Here we come to the practicalities – the techniques for going about it.

Although in deep meditation the mind is completely still and beyond technique, few people are able to slip into this state of stillness straight away. This is why we take the support of techniques to deal with the mind and the constant stream of thoughts, emotions and inner chatter that fill it. Fortunately sages have offered us countless different methods – such as breath-awareness techniques, mantras, visualization and awareness practices – which give the mind a focus and allow it to settle back into the inner spaciousness.

Deciding which technique to use can be time-consuming. To avoid wasting precious hours it helps to bear in mind that technique are not ends, but means, and that there is no 'right' or 'best' way. Unless you have been instructed in a particular practice by an enlightened teacher, in which case it may be empowered and yield quicker results, the best technique to start with is one you feel drawn to or that feels natural.

Practise your chosen technique for ten minutes once or twice a day. You can meditate at any time, but first thing in the morning, when your mind is at its clearest and most uncluttered, is ideal. Persevere for long enough – a week or two – to get a sense of how the practice affects you. If you feel calmer and more relaxed, and find it satisfying and enjoyable, keep on meditating using the technique. Meditation teaches you meditation, and once you have found a way that suits you it is beneficial to go more deeply into it, at least for a time, rather than continue experimenting. Finding it a struggle, however, is an indication that the practice is not right for you, at any rate for the moment, and you would probably gain more from experimenting with other methods. Only you can know what works best for you – meditation is a journey of discovery.

Meditation positions

Because they are very stable, the classic positions – the lotus and perfect postures (*see* below and on page 44) – are ideal for meditation, but if you are unable to sit in them comfortably for any length of time assume either a simple cross-legged position (*see* page 45) or sit on a straight-backed chair, keeping your back straight but relaxed. You can also meditate in the corpse position (*see* page 115), but beware of falling asleep.

Lotus

The lotus position, in which the Buddha is classically depicted, is the very symbol of meditation. The legs are locked together providing a stable base from which the meditator will neither topple over nor fall asleep, and no effort is required to maintain the position. Although it is very relaxing once hips, knees and ankles have become sufficiently flexible, the posture is invariably uncomfortable to begin with, particularly if you are accustomed only to sitting in a chair. Never force your legs into this position as doing so can damage the knee tendons.

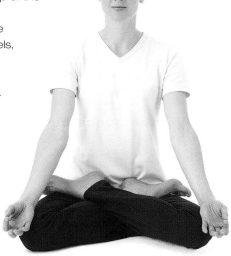

Instructions

1 Sit on the floor with your legs outstretched.
2 Bend your right knee and place the foot on the left thigh, heel pressing into the abdomen, sole upturned.
3 Bend your left knee and gently place the foot on top of the right thigh in a similar way.
4 Place your hands on your knees, palms up, with the thumb and first finger touching, or between the heels, one over the other.
5 Begin by holding the position for up to a minute, gradually increasing the length of time you stay in it.

Focus points

- In the classic lotus the left leg is placed on top, but to develop equal flexibility on both sides it is best to reverse the roles of the legs regularly. This applies to all cross-legged postures.

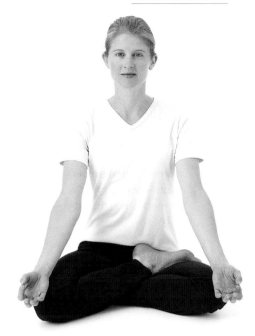

Half lotus

If you find it difficult to sit in the full lotus you may like to start with the half lotus.

Instructions

1 Sit on the floor with your legs outstretched.
2 Bend your left knee and place your left foot beneath the right thigh as close as possible to your buttocks.
3 Bend your right knee and place your right foot on top of the left thigh as in the full lotus. Both knees should touch the ground and the back should be kept straight.
4 Place your hands as for the full lotus and regularly reverse the positions of the legs.

Breath-awareness techniques

Focusing attention on the breath is an effective way of stilling the mind and many meditation techniques are built around it. These are natural techniques which most people feel comfortable with as they have no religious or philosophical connotations.

Following your breath

1 Sit in any crossed-legged position or on a chair keeping your back comfortably straight.
2 Close your eyes and breathe naturally, taking your attention to your breath as it comes in and goes out.
3 Become absorbed in the movement of the breath until you glide into meditation.
4 Whatever thoughts and feelings arise, just let them be without engaging with them. Gently bring your attention back to the breath.

Watching the space between breaths

Meditate as above, focusing on the space between breaths – the space in which the inhalation expires and before the exhalation arises, and the space outside where the exhalation expires and before the inhalation arises.

Counting breaths

Breathing naturally, meditate as described above in 'Following your breath', counting either the inhalations or the exhalations from one to ten, repeating the procedure throughout the meditation.

The *hamsa* (*so'ham*) technique

This is a simple technique of observing the breath as it flows in and out in combination with the *hamsa* mantra. According to yogic literature, the sound *hamsa* is continuously repeated by every living being, whether they are aware of it or not, and for this reason it is called the 'natural mantra'. The sequence *hamsa-hamsa-hamsa* can also be heard as *so'ham-so'ham-so'ham*, Sanskrit for 'I am that', when the order of the syllables is reversed.

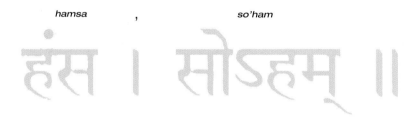

hamsa   ,   so'ham

हंस । सोऽहम् ॥

1 Sit in any crossed-legged position or on a chair keeping your back comfortably straight.
2 Close your eyes and breathe naturally, taking your attention to your breath as it comes in and goes out.
3 As you breathe in, hear the sound *ham* (pronounced *hum*) and as you breathe out, *sa* (*sah* or *so*). Focus your attention on the spaces between breaths – between *ham* and *sa*, and between *sa* and *ham*.
4 Whatever thoughts and feelings arise, just let them be without engaging with them. Simply bring your attention back to the breath and awareness of the mantra.
5 Once you experience the stillness in the centre of your being, let go of the *ham* and the *sa* and lose yourself in meditation.

Mantra meditation

Silent repetition of a mantra is the most popular form of meditation. A mantra is a sacred or mystical sound, syllable or word said to possess spiritual potency that affects the consciousness of the person who repeats it. The most famous of all mantras is *om* (composed of the three sounds *a-u-m*), which is said to be the primordial sound from which the entire universe arises. Other mantras are often preceded by *om*, such as *om mani padme hum*, '*om*, the jewel in the lotus', much used by Tibetan Buddhists, and *om namah shivaya*, a traditional Indian mantra honouring Shiva. According to esoteric tradition, however, a mantra will bear spiritual fruit and lead to heightened states of consciousness only when empowered by and received from an enlightened teacher.

However that may be, for the purposes of deep relaxation a meaningless word or sound will do just as well. Choose any word or sound that appeals to you, the shorter the better, or use a positive word, phrase or affirmation, or even your own name. Once you have found a mantra, word or sound you feel comfortable with, stick with it and use it at odd moments during the day to relax you.

• Of all mantras, the most celebrated is the sacred syllable *om*. Its symbolic representation, shown here, is often used as a focus of visual meditation.

1 Sit in any crossed-legged position or on a chair keeping your back comfortably straight.
2 Close your eyes and breathe naturally.
3 Repeat your chosen mantra, word or sound silently at a normal speaking rate, and preferably in rhythm with your breathing – once or twice as you breath in, once or twice as you breathe out. Focus your attention on the mantra and become absorbed in it.
4 Whatever thoughts and feelings arise, observe them passively. Let them be without engaging with them and gently bring your attention back to your mantra.

Visual meditation

This kind of meditation involves gazing steadily at an object such as a lighted candle, a flower or a symbol of spiritual or religious significance such as the Christian cross, the yin-yang symbol or a yantra, which is the visual equivalent of a mantra (*see* above). A lighted candle in a darkened room is a popular choice because the eyes are naturally drawn to the brightness of the flame, and the image is easy to retain when the eyes are closed.

1 Sit in any crossed-legged position or on a chair keeping your back comfortably straight, having placed your chosen object between three and six feet away from you and roughly level with your eyes.

2 Breathing naturally, focus your attention on the object and gaze at it in a steady, relaxed way, without staring, and blinking as usual whenever you need to.

3 When your eyes tire close them and form a mental image of your chosen object.

4 If you become aware that you have lost concentration, or that your attention has wandered, gently bring it back to your meditation focus. If necessary repeat the process of gazing at it, then visualizing it with your mind's eye.

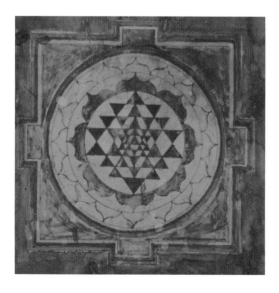

• The Shri Yantra is one of the most celebrated of all mandalas. It represents the yogic vision of the cosmos and the evolutionary process, and is often used in meditation to draw the yoga practitioner inwards.

golden rules

- Stop smoking

- Protect your skin from the sun

- Meditate

- Get plenty of sleep

- Make time to relax

- Maintain good posture, sitting or standing

- Take regular, moderate exercise

- Eat more fruit and vegetables – at least five portions a day

- Drink at least two litres of water a day

- Have regular health and dental checks

- Learn to manage stress

- Do not constantly talk about your health or problems

- Look on the bright side – optimists live longer

- Spend time with young people

- Be proactive – make new friends, do voluntary work

- Have more sex (within a loving relationship)

- Keep informed and up to date

- Be creative, daydream

- Learn new skills and be open to new experiences

- Accept yourself, and what you cannot change about yourself

- Develop your sense of humour

- Smile and laugh a lot

- Don't give in to anyone's preconceptions about ageing – be defiant

- Don't take yourself too seriously

- Above all, don't take anti-ageing too seriously. Life's too short!

acknowledgements

The idea for 10-Minute Anti-Ageing arose during a conversation with Camilla Stoddart of Cassell Illustrated, who immediately saw its potential and reacted fast. Many thanks for your enthusiasm, encouragement and perspicacious comments on the text. I am also grateful to the entire Cassell team for their support and vital contribution to the book, and most particularly to Victoria Alers-Hankey for her editorial eye and deft juggling of text and illustrations to fit, Austin Taylor for his painstaking work in creating an attractive and user-friendly design, and Jo Knowles for a great cover. Thanks once again to Paul Bricknell for the great shots of Jo Robertson (46), Jan Mortimer (44) and Sandi Sharkey (37), and to all of them for modelling so beautifully.

I could not have written this book without the inspiration and contribution of many un-Botoxed, uncosmetically treated, unsurgically enhanced 30, 40 and 50-something women who have generously shared the secrets of their sensational and youthful good looks. My grateful thanks to all and especially to Sarah Whitehead, Becky Viney and Jane Ross-Macdonald for their help and expertise. Jo Robertson of Yogabase, the Islington yoga studio, deserves a special mention and tremendous thanks for her invaluable contribution. As well as modelling for the photos, she devised the anti-gravity exercise sequences without which this book would be incomplete. As the illustrations show she is a shining example of just how much can be achieved with them.

Meditation has played a vital role in my life and informed my approach to anti-ageing. I first noticed its youth-enhancing effects many years ago, and am pleased to find that research has confirmed these early observations. I am most grateful to the exceptional teachers I have been privileged to know and learn from, and above all to Baba Muktananda, late guru of the Siddha yoga tradition, who set alight the fire of meditation within me and fanned the flame in a most extraordinary way.

Last but not least, fond thanks to my wonderful family, especially my mother Thorven for her insights into ageing, love and unflagging support; my uncle Philip Cranford-Smith for professional advice and for being living proof that it is possible to look great, be on the ball and have a life in your seventies; and my remarkable husband, the publisher Nicholas Brealey, and our son Sam for love, laughs and a constant supply of cuddles. Best thanks go to Sam who has just told me I look about 26!